Dear Marin

Can Marin County Reach the United Nations
Sustainable Development Goals of 2030?
A Systems Thinking Perspective

FELICIA I. CHAVEZ, PhD, MBA

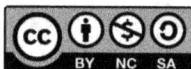

To Elberta & Ricardo...
...who inspire me. Without whom my work in Marin
would have been far less effective, and far more boring.

To Tricia...
...who believes in me. Without whom my work in
Marin would not have been possible.

Contents

DEAR MARIN

Preface

Dear Marin,

I'm leaving. Having been born and raised in Northern California, it's time I spend at least a period of time living far away, perhaps even overseas. However, as I have been directly involved since 2017 in local attempts to make Marin County a better place, I want to leave you with my notes, in a manner of speaking. I have been to many, oh-so-many meetings, and one of the things I have learned is that local residents of Marin are vastly underinformed about the real social and ecological state of our very own place.

I presume you, the reader, are a fan of Marin County, but also, that you would like to see some things change. You feel uncomfortable about the fact that Marin is mostly White and highly economically and racially segregated, but you also feel underqualified to meaningfully help. You know you could do a better job saving energy and putting more veggies in your diet, but there's only so much a person can fit in a day. You're concerned about climate change, but the details on how to *really* make a *significant* difference are fuzzy. You care about helping people, particularly women and girls, and suspect there are things you could be doing in your own community, aside from volunteering on the occasional event committee and making monetary donations or charity auction item purchases.

In short, you'd like to think of yourself as someone willing to get her hands dirty to help save the world, but it's just not clear where to start, if what you *are* doing is enough, or if the organizations you support are making a meaningful impact. What is the reality behind those shiny, up-beat annual reports and appeals?

This book is for you.

Many of us think that Marin County is special. In terms of our geography and some really nice natural areas, we *are* special; certainly, unique.

However, when it comes to our *society*, I'm afraid we are merely a symptom of the larger whole: extreme and worsening income inequality, structural and social racism (both covert and overt), gender discrimination, and a totally dramatically *un*-sustainable way of life, courtesy of our cradle-to-grave economy.

It doesn't have to be this way.

In addition to some first-hand stories, I do my best to "translate" from reports that are often not very user-friendly, written by specialists for specialists (and often for much larger geographic regions). Usually these reports are lost in nonprofit website archives or lingering in boxes in the back of a board member's closet. I also draw from community group conversations (and their endless easel pad transcriptions), and conversations with Marin residents from a variety of backgrounds.

As a promoter of systems thinking, I am constantly seeking ways for us to "help the system to become conscious of itself" (to reference Otto Scharmer and Theory U). As a community organizer since 2017—and Marin resident since 1995—I can tell you that Marin County is largely *not* conscious of itself. This lack of community-wide consciousness is a problem for our whole society, well beyond Marin, and it is at the root of our profound non-sustainability, whether we're talking people, planet, or prosperity.

That is why I took the time to put this book together *for you*.

The way forward requires a lot of work, but not necessarily *new* work. Rather, what is required is a new perspective brought to the same work we are already doing. This new way needs to be collaborative, coordinated, and caring.

Unfortunately, the way philanthropy is structured, organizations are forced to compete with each other rather than collaborate, hobbled by linear check-box-style "impact" reporting. Important individual activists are overlooked and underfunded, particularly if they don't have a 501(c)(3) entity in which to contextualize themselves.

And for those who *are* registered 501(c)(3) organizations, they too are often overlooked or underfunded. According to TaxExemptWorld.com, there are 4,186 registered nonprofits in Marin.[1] With almost 260,000 people, that's about one NGO per 60 people in Marin. While many of these organizations are not doing local work, a good handful of them are, and they are forced to compete for your attention through the din of national, and even global media and advertising.

I invite you to see our county through the eyes of one person who has spent over half of her life in Marin. I invite you

---

1   "Marin County California Nonprofits and 501c Organizations - Search and Download Lists," Tax Exempt World, March 26, 2022, https://www.taxexemptworld.com/organizations/marin-county-ca-california.asp.

to try on a systems view. I have crafted this text such that by the end you are far more informed, and your worldview is a bit more flexible, inclusive, and sharp. After that, I hope you come back to me with better insights than are perhaps found herein, informed by your own thoughtfulness, experiences, and sincere desire to contribute positively to our world.

Introduction

Europeans have inhabited Marin County for hardly 200 years, but the society that sprang from European immigration is already endangered, in small and large ways. Youth, elders, and low or even moderate-income people can't afford to live here. According to the Environmental Working Group (EWG), our drinking water is just-maybe-ok: their tests cite 24 total contaminants in Marin Municipal Water District tap water, with 12 exceeding EWG's health guidelines.[2] According to the Marin Convention and Visitor's Bureau, this county has set aside nearly 85% of our land for preservation.[3] However, much of that land is insufficiently tended, building up fuel that constitutes catastrophic wildfires-waiting-to-happen. And we haven't even begun to discuss the threats climate change poses to low-lying areas, of which we have many.

We could address our challenges far more comprehensively and sustainably than we currently are. Many individuals and organizations are working on those challenges. **They just aren't yet working together to the degree necessary to be actually effective.**

---

2   "Marin Municipal Water District," Environmental Working Group, 2020, https://www.ewg.org/tapwater/system.php?pws=CA2110002?pws=CA2110002.

3   "The Bay and Protected Open Space," Marin County Convention and Visitors Bureau, accessed August 25, 2022, https://www.visitmarin.org/things-to-do/outdoor-activities/the-bay-and-protected-open-space/.

"Working together" entails a whole lot of interpersonal progress. Bickering, irritability, territoriality, half-truths, niceness over truthiness, and flat-out undermining other groups or organizations is our Achilles heel (true for our whole society, I might add). And coordination is not enough: we need *synergy*.

If you're anything like me, you have seen far too many documentaries about horrible threats and dire warnings about the future of life on Earth. Maybe you have started eating a more plant-based diet, driving less, buying less, flying less, growing more food, and donating more. But it never quite feels like enough. That's because **it isn't**. There is nothing easy about "being green," despite the slick advertisements to the contrary. And it's *even harder* to be socially just, given current economic systems. As long as you feel like it's just you and a handful of "like-minded people," it's never going to be enough. A completely different approach—one both new and old—is necessary.

These issues are anything but linear; anything but easy and obvious. Relationships among the various issues are many, hidden, and tangled.

A Personal Anecdote

One afternoon, in approximately 2002, I was sitting at my desk in the reception area of an environmental nonprofit in Oakland, California. Something unusual was happening in me that day.

Out of the clear blue sky, I had a persistent, nagging need to be outside, in nature, among trees. And I knew exactly where I wanted to be: at the base of the Cataract Trail, near Cataract Falls, situated at a far corner of Alpine Lake in Marin County.

I finally managed to extract myself from my sense of duty that would normally keep me in my seat until 5:00. I raced (within lawful limits) the hour-and-a-quarter it took to get to my desired spot. I had an appointment back at my house in San Rafael at 6:00 (a friend was helping me fix my recalcitrant computer), so I would have precious little time to immerse myself in the trees.

Over the Richmond-San Rafael bridge, out Sir Francis Drake, through Fairfax and over the hill, past the Alpine dam. . . I parked at the base of the trail and met the destination that had called to me at my desk in downtown Oakland: the trail with the trees, the water, the air.

Walking along the compact dirt trail, I reflected that I only had ten minutes or so before I'd have to drive the 45 minutes back to my house in San Rafael.

Believe it or not, it was totally worth it. I was in desperate need of this environment. Absorbing the energy of the forest, I walked slowly, feeling the living foliage, reaching out with my fingertips to physically acknowledge the Green, contemplating with wonder the lessening of the barrier I normally felt between me and the natural environment. "Wow," I thought to myself, "I must have *really* needed this."

Marin County

Whenever I tell San Francisco Bay Area residents I live in Marin, their invariable response is, "Marin? It's so *beautiful* there. You're very lucky to live in such a beautiful place." In other words, the hallmark of this place is, in fact, its natural beauty.

I imagine that many people throughout the Bay Area have experienced that utterly profound sense of *green life* that I experienced that day on the trail, or they are at least drawn in that direction for some deeper reason they may or may not be able to articulate.

Marin embodies the experience of proximity to nature that is a profound service to our whole region. It's not just ecosystem services Marin provides, it's psychological, emotional, and spiritual support services, even for people who don't come here, they *know* Marin is here, and believe it or not, that may help someone get through the day.

Marin features a small but dignified mountain, Tamalpais, the Bay on one side, the Pacific on the other, and ancient Redwood trees and stately elk and all kinds of flora and fauna in between.

There was no Bay Area master plan that designated Marin County should henceforth be largely preserved so that all other Bay Area residents would have a great place to visit. (At least, not that I know of.) Much of Marin was slated for development until resident activists intervened, dedicating whole lifetimes to protecting and preserving large areas of land. Thus, residents, and people far and near have the opportunity to enjoy the open spaces, parks, views, hiking, biking, horseback riding, camping, birding, etc.

But this abundance of open spaces comes with a cost, and as is typical in human civilization, it is low-income groups who first and foremost bear the burden.

When I made that spur-of-the-moment trip back to Marin to fill my nature-lover-energy bank, I had only recently moved back to Marin after living just on the other side of Highway 37 for three years, in Vallejo. After graduating from Dominican University in San Rafael in 1999, my roommate and I could *not* find an affordable place to live. So, for three years I slept at our affordable condo in Vallejo, worked in Oakland, and spent the rest of my time in Marin County. My bank, car mechanic, boyfriend, grocery stores, friends, odd jobs, alma matter, and all matters of other life preoccupations were located here, in Marin.

The United Nations Sustainable Development Goals

Let's zoom to the global view, and explore why and how the Global Goals are relevant locally. To help us get a handle on the complexity of interweaving challenges already described, the first six United Nations Sustainable Development Goals (SDGs) of 2030 serve as the organizing framework of this book. This conundrum of feeling like you are not doing enough, and not enough people around you are doing enough, is largely a symptom of not having a framework like the SDGs in widespread usage here locally.

As you may know, a lot of people *are* doing a *lot*. I'm sure you, like me, get pounds of mail, dozens of emails (and dozens of social media mentions) about groups doing all kinds of things. But they are not doing it together, in coordination with government, corporations, residents and other NGOs, so we're nowhere near sufficiently visible to one another, nor sufficiently effective.

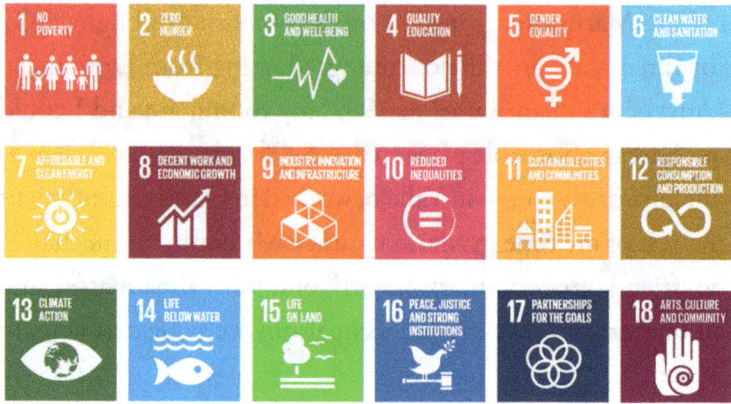

Figure 1 - United Nations Sustainable Development Goals of 2030

The first six SDGs are the organizing framework of this book. I chose to go in-depth with this first set rather than doing a briefer look at all the Global Goals.

Note that I have added an 18th Goal to the original seventeen: "Arts, Culture, and Community." This is a key area for perhaps all SDGs: without a rich arts landscape and a powerful sense of community we are ill equipped to make any meaningful progress toward common aims.

Some topics aren't covered by the SDGs; for example, animal rights. Still, I find them pretty darn handy. Also, setting society-wide (much less worldwide) goals is something we haven't done much of. President John F. Kennedy set a space exploration goal for the decade of the 1960's, and some nations have set goals in recent history. But here in the U.S., it's less common. (So-called "campaign promises" seem to have taken up the room that specific, measurable goals would otherwise occupy.)

Each of the Global Goals has a set of targets underneath it. So for example, SDG #1 "No Poverty" lists seven targets (or five targets and two additional ones labeled "A" and "B"), such as 1.1 "By 2030, eradicate extreme poverty for all people everywhere. . . "[4] I reference these targets in each chapter.

While the SDGs are the doorway in, they are also merely symbolic of a vastly complex reality. That is why we need systems thinking: our navigational guide for complexity. More on systems thinking later.

It is powerful for Marin County as a society to ask ourselves, for example, "What do we as a county want to see by December of 2030 with regard to #1 No Poverty? How do we define poverty?" and similar questions on down the list for all of the Goals. If our purpose is being a nice place for relatively wealthy families to live and raise kids, the answer to this question is *different* than if our purpose is health and well-being for actually-really everyone. Unfortunately, as the following chapters will detail, we are behaving as if our purpose is the former. (We will discuss this idea of "purpose" from a "systems thinking" perspective in more depth later.) All number of NGOs, government agencies and community groups work to make up the gap, but the gap continues to widen in many, if not most cases.

---

4   UNDP, "Goal 1 End Poverty in All Its Forms Everywhere," United Nations Sustainable Development, August 25, 2022, https://www. un.org/sustainabledevelopment/poverty/.

Our Local Native North American Groups–
Coast Miwok

Native American individuals *are* present in Marin County. But due to the small number of individuals, they are usually left out of community reports and studies entirely. While on the one hand this is due to the nuances of the nature of data, privacy, and statistics, on the other, it subliminally sends the message to readers that there are no Native people present in a given group, and it may leave a Native person with the impression that they don't matter. As we go through each of the Global Goals, I cite limited available data about the quality of life experienced by Native North Americans generally ("American Indians and Alaska Natives"), and peoples native to California where possible. In particular SDG #5 Gender Equality includes an extended look at the plight of Native North American women.

Systems Thinking

Compared to the SDGs, systems thinking is not limited to a "field," rather, it is an entire worldview. I'm going to make two claims here that I don't think you should *believe*, but rather, *entertain* in the context of this book.

1. In the United States, we are brought up in ways that heavily reinforce a linear, reductionist, analytical worldview. We are good at looking closely, at pulling things apart, at reducing them to their component parts.

a. The systems worldview—or, seeing the world as a great web of interconnected relationships—is not supported, and usually, actively driven out.

2. Systems thinking is **required** in order to create a sustainable world. Until we can *think* like an ecosystem, we can't build our society like a resilient ecosystem.

The half-hour "Systems Thinking Mini-Course" on the Systems Thinking Marin website provides you with a video version of these basic principles:

1. Systems thinking means attending to relationships
2. Systems thinking requires changing your default perspective
3. Systems thinking enables you to hold the one and the many

Note, however, that these are not exclusive categories. They are deeply and inherently intertwined. Let us begin with #1, "Relationships."

Relationships

This means relationships between humans, between humans and the environment, between species and their environment, and even between abstract principles.

When you are focusing linearly, you attend to points. When you are looking at a system, you attend to relationships; the spaces in between. Points are quantifiable; relationships are qualities (i.e., "qualitative").

Much of this text relies on data points, but when we talk about positive change, we need to bring in the relationships aspect, the qualities. Relationships come up repeatedly in the two remaining sections below: "Change Your Default Perspective" and the "Hold the One and the Many."

Change Your Default Perspective

This means shifting your default way of planning and doing thusly:

- From short-term to long-term
- From narrow to wide
- From shallow or surface to deep

And sometimes, from a focus on what's happening externally to a focus on what is happening internally; from looking for the causes of a situation *out there* to looking at *my role* in making the world a better or worse place.

These perspective shifts are relative to where you are starting from. For an example of short to long-term, let's say you are a small animal rights organization working on your strategic plan for three years into the future. A long-term plan for you to consider is twenty years out. A systems view calls for this longer-term thinking.

If, however, you are a local government agency, a ten-year plan is a starting place. As a government, you are responsible for attending to people throughout their whole lifetime, and the next generation, and the next. . . A hundred-year plan forces issues of social and ecological sustainability; a ten-year plan does not. If your agency is not planning for the long-term picture of our society, no one is.

See the book *The Good Ancestor: A Radical Prescription for Long-Term Thinking* by Roman Krznaric, for more details on long-term thinking.

In addition to the references later in this text, I will leave it to you to consider what "narrow to wide" and "shallow or surface to deep" looks like. Again, these are as much "felt qualities" as they are quantifiable.

Hold the One & the Many

My favorite example of systems thinking is astrology. Even if you don't give a hoot about astrology, it's a brain-challenging exercise to contemplate, say, a natal chart. "You see, your sun is in the first house on the ascendant, aspected to your Pluto in the third, trine your Venus. . . " Holding all of those planets and aspects and *feeling* their relationships—their qualities— gives you an immediate sense of what "holding the one and the many" requires.

Or take an ecosystem example. The owl hunts the small mammal, so if you as the human in the situation install a thoughtfully built and appropriately located (all of which are systems questions) owl box, you just might have friendly neighborhood help with keeping rats out of your garden. But if your neighbor puts out rodent poison and the owl gets ahold of the poisoned rodent, your ally is compromised, perhaps killed. If you have a good relationship with your neighbor, you may be able to discuss your hopes, dreams, and property needs with them. If not, perhaps not.

All of these factors are ever-changing parts of dynamic systems that influence one another. We cannot reasonably hope to consciously synthesize all factors (known and unknown) and realistically calculate the chances of each factor going in our favor, especially because the combination of a multitude of factors creates systems dynamics that are even more complex. However, we can "get a feel" for a situation. Rather than attempting to control every aspect through analytical calculations (and freaking out or blaming others when things go awry), we have the option in complex situations to move into the complexity "holding" the one and the many as we go in a spirit of opening.

Relationships - Again

The major systems focal point in this book is relationships, though all three of these factors discussed above are deeply intertwined. I have separated them out for purposes of discussion. Seek opportunities to see into the depth of relationship between these three perspectives.

Systems Thinking: Not for Every Situation

Note that systems thinking is not appropriate for every situation in life. There is a useful framework called the *Cynefin* (a Welsh word) created by Dave Snowden that helps you to understand and differentiate when a systems versus a more conventional (i.e., "linear") approach is called for.

In brief, if there is *a right answer* that *can* be known ahead of time, you're in the realm of the linear. If you are a human resources officer dealing with making sure your employees go through their government mandated sexual harassment training, your attempts to get them to complete the training may be helped by some systems principles, but essentially you are working to check some regulatory boxes. If, however, your organization has a recurrent problem of sexual harassment and you're working to change internal culture, that's when you need systems thinking.

I heard an example at a training a while back that provided this example. If you know there are some young women graduating from high school in your neighborhood who have college aspirations but are short of college funds, helping to organize the neighborhood to start a fundraising campaign to help them is a fairly straight-forward approach that calls for linear tools. Yes of course, your relationships come into play here but essentially, you have identified a funding gap, and you are moved to help close that gap.

If, however, you want to tackle the issue of college being out of reach for lower income (and these days, middle income) families, that is a complex situation, and therefore calls for systems thinking.

Money & Systems

In 2016, I attended the Marin Equity Summit. During the afternoon breakout session, I looked around the room at the various tables with their group labels and wondered if maybe-perhaps there would be an "Interstitial Space" or "Overlapping Issues" table. No such luck. So, I defaulted to the Economics and Jobs table, because when you're lacking a systems level group the Economics table is the next best thing.

You will note repeatedly that funding—no surprise here— underlies social and ecological outcomes. That would seem like common sense. However, despite the prevalence of collo- quialisms such as "Follow the money," we often fail to actually do that. When you follow the money you by default are almost always taking a systems perspective. Currency *flows*. Access and privilege follow money. In the chapters that follow, again and again attending to the presence or absence of money gives us an inside view of just what the heck is going on. Money, and access to it, matters.

"Sustainable Development" & Systems Thinking

As noted above, the chapters of this book are organized according to the "United Nations Sustainable Development Goals of 2030." This is a mouthful. Most people are plenty fuzzy on what precisely the U.N. does, much less the jargon of "sustainable development." Let's reference a brilliant systems thinker, Donella "Dana" Meadows, for help.

In a late 1990's talk (thank you to the person who kindly posted this on YouTube), Meadows references Herman Daly and Karl-Henrik Robèrt for a detailed definition of sustain- ability. What you see below is Donella's summary of their definition of "sustainable." It is the most comprehensive *and* easiest-to-understand definition I have come across (and I have an MBA in sustainable enterprise, so I've seen a lot of definitions).

Every RENEWABLE RESOURCE must be used at or below the rate at which it can regenerate itself. [For example, trees should not be cut down faster than they can grow back.]

Every NONRENEWABLE RESOURCE must be used at or below the rate at which a renewable substitute can be developed. [For instance, oil should not be used up faster than we can come up with alternatives.]

Every POLLUTION STREAM must be emitted at or below the rate at which it can be absorbed or made harmless. [So, if we are washing plastics out to sea, we should not be seeing them showing up later, in any form, or we need to stop that.]

To be SOCIALLY SUSTAINABLE, capital stocks and resource flows must be EQUITABLY DISTRIBUTED and SUFFICIENT to provide a good life for everyone. [This means no one goes hungry or homeless. No one.][5]

Meadows then goes on to say that none of our current systems are sustainable, from the organic farm she lives on, to the whole human socio-economic system of Earth.

The challenge my roommate and I faced in 1999 when we found ourselves living in Vallejo was a symptom of the

---

5   Jennifer Lynn, "Dana (Donella) Meadows Lecture: Sustainable Systems
     (Part 1 of 4)," YouTube, May 8, 2013, https://www.youtube.com/
     watch?v=HMmChiLZZHg.

collective cost of keeping Marin beautiful, and single-fami-
ly-home-neighborhood-centric. But lack of affordable housing
for the young (and elderly, and low-income) is only one part of
the price we are paying.

The Purpose of Marin County

Due to the hard work of environmentalists over decades, the
presence of MCE (formerly "Marin Clean Energy"), the recent
addition of municipal composting, and the historic presence
of hippies, you may have the mistaken impression that Marin
County is already doing everything we can—or at least, a lot—
to help. This is not true. These measures are, as they say, good
first steps, but not remotely enough. We are a symptom of a
larger, profoundly unsustainable economic system.

And that brings us to the question at the heart of this book:
What is the *purpose* of Marin County? This is a powerful question one can pose about any system, and again, is derived from
the work of Donella Meadows.

Marin County has some hint of a purpose beyond just
subsuming the same purpose as that of the global market
economy; the purpose of the latter being the growth of profit.
Maybe being beautiful and full of nature *is* the purpose. But
increasingly, the purpose seems to be providing a pleasant
backdrop for individuals and families in the upper echelons of
that global market economy: a safe place for wealthy families,
complete with lots of recreational space, relatively clean air,
nice views, large homes, and good schools.

Maybe that's fine; maybe it makes sense in the grand scheme
of things for Marin County to specifically be a place for

wealthy people to live. But I contend, from a systems thinking perspective, that even if the majority of citizens in the county agreed on this purpose, the laws of nature won't permit such homogeneity to persist for long. Diversity equals resilience, and homogenous income level is a particularly unsustainable form of homogeneity.

In any case, it's a fantasy that this purpose would be satisfactory if consciously, publicly considered. Wealthy people don't enjoy sitting in the traffic generated by people having to drive in from far-flung, but more affordable communities, any more than non-wealthy people do. And in any case, wealthy or not, no one is going to be able to live here when the waters rise and knock out sewage treatment and other public services that are largely located in the lowlands. Roads, hospitals, stores, police and fire stations... the people who staff and maintain those facilities won't be in a position to drive to Marin County to deal with them in the midst of a disaster.

For these reasons and many more, I contend that the purpose of Marin County should be human well-being.

From my perspective, human well-being fundamentally requires environmental well-being. And vice versa, if we can't get the human part right, the environment will continue to suffer.

Just imagine for a moment the possibility of our county deciding that human well-being is a worthy and noble purpose. Where would we look for guidance on how to judge when a decision is in support of well-being, and when a decision acts against this collective aspiration? Enter the SDGs.

Wealth Does Not Equal Well-Being

A brief note here: many people make a massive, catastrophic mistake presuming that "wealth" more or less equates to "well-being." A brief internet search for "wealth as a risk factor" reveals that this assumption couldn't be more flawed. Statistically speaking, the middle class have a better shot at well-being than poor or wealthy individuals and families. For example, LiveScience.com cited a study published in 2017 that claimed the following:

> *Overall, the study found higher rates of drinking to the point of intoxication and the use of pot among the wealthier students than among kids in the general U.S. population. Rich kids had rates that were at least double the national U.S. average for taking stimulant drugs, such as Adderall or Ritalin, as well as for experimenting with cocaine. . .* [6]

As I learned from Don Carney, Executive Director of Youth Transforming Justice, money equals access, including access to substances. For more information, check out the classic book *The Golden Ghetto: The Psychology of Affluence.*

---

6   Carl Nierenberg, "Rich Kids and Drugs: Addiction May Hit Wealthy Students Hardest," Live Science, June 1, 2017, https://www.livescience. com/59329-drug-alcohol-addiction-wealthy-students.html.

The Work Required to Reach the Global Goals

Before we get into the individual SDG chapters, here I supply you with some important pieces that are referenced throughout this book. Note that in editing this book the upcoming section was a bit of a challenge. It's a little bit like in Buddhism where you have the five-this and eight-that and four-this, etc. Let me try to set this up clearly.

First, I present two models. After that, I supply you with a set of steps, "Stepping Toward Change," that apply to every "How Do We Get There?" section of the upcoming chapters.

1. The first model has three layers, like a cake, and I created it.
2. The second model has six levels (in this version) and I borrow it from Donella Meadows.
3. The third piece is not a model, but rather, as mentioned, a set of suggested steps, of which there are 12.

The first two, the models, are referred to here and there throughout *Dear Marin*, and are important for understanding the larger picture; of what is at work when we look out at our society and see that things are not working out well for many people. With regard to the suggested steps, rather than repeating them at the end of each chapter, they are supplied here once, and are meant to be loose; left up to interpretation and adaptation.

We begin with the first of the two models, the three-layer cake.

Charitable, Advocacy, Systems

You can use the model below to differentiate between three different levels of focus in local systems, particularly among nonprofit organizations trying to help people or the environment.

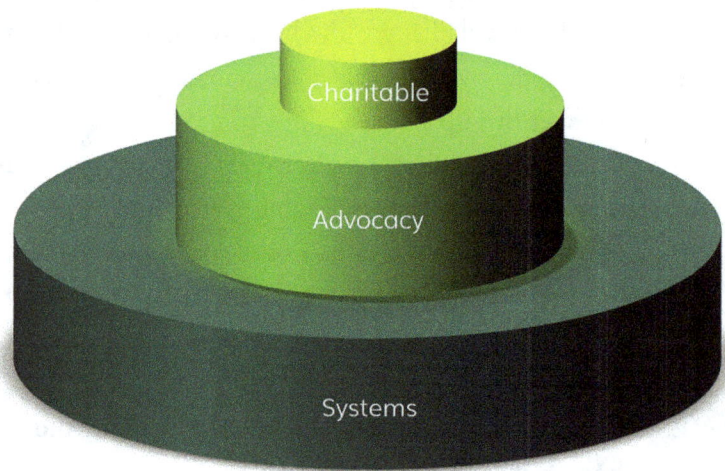

Figure 2 - Levels of Focus in a System

Charitable or Direct Service Level

Organizations that fall into the category of "Charitable or Direct Service" constitute what you would normally think of when someone mentions "nonprofits." They are the heroes who are there to catch people (or families, or species, or landscapes) before they are lost, whether due to human activity or natural disasters. While they make up the bulk of NGOs, here they are presented visually as "the tip of the iceberg." They are the wildlife hospitals like WildCare in San Rafael, the Earth First'ers blocking bulldozers, the job training programs, the emergency cash to cover utilities, and even financial aid for education and pretty much anything you might think of as "welfare services" or "social services." Examples include the San Francisco–Marin Food Bank, MarinLink's "Warm Wishes" program (backpacks of supplies for homeless individuals during the cold months), and a tutoring program at your local school.

Advocacy Level

These are the people who show up at city council meetings, who write letters, meet with and lobby policy makers, march in the streets, and who work to inform their neighbors. They are attempting to improve existing systems; to get the existing system to *do something different*. Though there are not as many advocacy groups as there are charitable organizations, they are out there, and you are likely familiar with at least a few of them. Examples include the Bay Area Industrial Areas Foundation/Marin Organizing Committee, and 350 Marin. (Many local advocacy organizations are locally-run chapters of national organizations.)

Systems Level

This level is presented as the largest, lowest layer of the cake to represent that it underlies everything else. Systems-level groups are nearly nonexistent. This should be where government operates, but for a variety of reasons, it does not. The simplest versions are simply round-tables that allow participants in a local community to gather regularly. Here people build relationships and share news and resources. I have supported two of these efforts in Marin City between 2017 and 2022, Elberta Erkisson's Southern Marin Multi-Disciplinary Team, and Ricardo Moncrief's ISOJI group.

Here is an example of taking the systems level to the extreme. It is a grim one—and national as opposed to local—but it will serve to illustrate what it looks like to operate at this level. Through it you can see that "systems thinking" does not equal "virtuous." Rather, the tools of systems thinking can be used to make the world a worse place. And, we can learn from the strategy of the evil ones, as it were.

The book *Dark Money: The Hidden History of the Billionaires Behind the Rise of the Radical Right* by Jane Mayer, profiles the extremist Libertarian billionaire version of systems level intervention.

> *During the 1970s, a handful of the nation's wealthiest corporate captains felt overtaxed and overregulated and decided to fight back. Disenchanted with the direction of modern America, they launched an ambitious, privately financed war of ideas to radically change the country. They didn't want to merely win elections; they wanted to change how Americans thought. Their ambitions were grandiose—to "save" America as they saw it, at every level, by turning the clock back to the Gilded Age before the advent of the Progressive Era.*[7]

---

7   Jane Mayer, Dark Money: How a Secretive Group of Billionaires Is Trying to Buy Political Control in the US (London: Scribe Publications, 2016), 461.

Some have called this cabal the "Kochtopus," in reference to the Koch brothers at the center of the effort. In reality, their strategy ran the gamut from systems to advocacy to direct intervention. The key here, however, is that their direct and advocacy levels were deeply informed by, and coordinated with, their systems level worldview and strategy.

Systems level interventions are certainly not always multi-billion-dollar undertakings over decades. However, to be effective, they do need to be hooked up to the advocacy and charitable/direct service work that takes place further downstream. And in addition, the charitable/direct service and advocacy levels are most effective when the systems part of the structure is included. One might argue that efforts to make the world a better place lack effectiveness and largely fail due to a profound absence of this multi-tiered cooperation and alignment.

Local examples of a systems level approach include the Novato City Council taking the lead in Marin County to raise their minimum wage (with the direct involvement of the organization North Bay Jobs With Justice). Another example is Marin Community Foundation's experimental universal basic income program for low-income mothers in Marin.

However, the deepest systems work in Marin—and anywhere in North America—requires us to look at the role of Native North Americans in the ecology of this land. Based on my limited knowledge in this regard, I propose that it would be difficult if not impossible to find a species of indigenous plant or animal here in Marin that local peoples did *not* have some kind of involved, functional relationship with. (I'll refer you to the book *Tending the Wild* by M. Kat Anderson for more information.) The opposite is true of most of us living in Marin today.

The Hierarchy of Intervention

Turning back to Donella Meadows, she supplies us with a model for thinking about where to intervene in a system. I call this the "Hierarchy of Intervention." See the image below for my version of a slide Meadows presents at one of her talks. The uppermost level, "Mindset or Worldview," is the place with the greatest leverage or potential for change in a system, but it is also most difficult to change. The lowest level, "Events," gives you basically zero leverage, but is easiest to change.

Mindsets / Worldviews

⬇

Function / Purpose / Goal

⬇

Interconnections / Relationships

⬇

Elements

⬇

Behavior

⬇

The nightly news

Events

Adapted from: "Dana (Donella) Meadows Lecture: Sustainable Systems (Part 3 of 4)," YouTube.

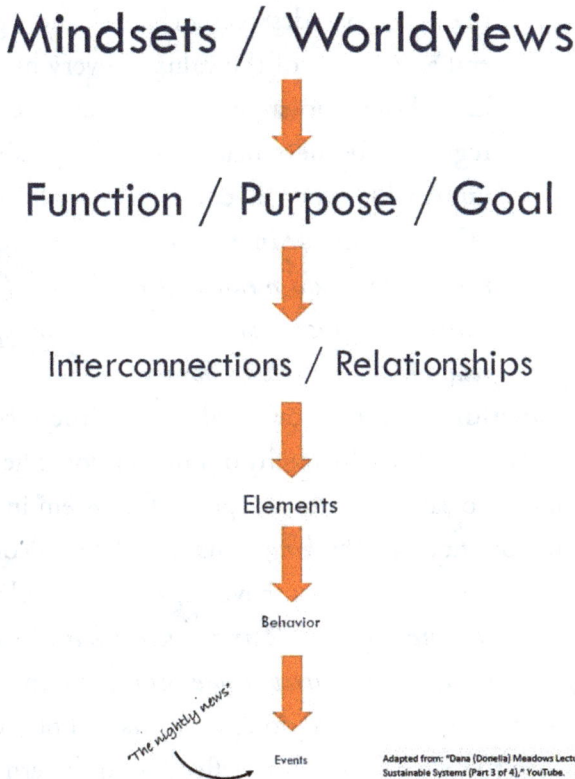

Figure 3 - Meadow's "Leverage Points to Intervene in a System" or "Hierarchy of Intervention"

1. **Mindset or Worldviews**: This is the very top of the hierarchy. Changing mindset or worldviews is the place of greatest leverage for downstream change. However, it's also the toughest to change.

   a. Example: Consider immigration of Central and South American people at the southern border of the United States. Those who support open borders may have the perspective that "everyone deserves a chance" and a general acceptance of the value of every human life. Those who support closed and heavily regulated borders place other things above human life when it comes to people from other countries. *Intervening at the level of worldview would mean shifting the belief system(s) that causes a person to support or oppose relatively open or closed borders.*

2. **Function, Purpose, or Goal**: This is the second tier in Meadows' hierarchy of intervention. She has much to say about the purpose of a system in her important book *Thinking in Systems.* When it comes to human systems, you have to, as she articulates, *stand around for a while and watch what a system produces to discern its purpose.* Often the people within a given system don't know its real purpose: they too have to do some reflecting to discern the purpose.

   a. To take the Southern U.S. border immigration example, we would ask something like, "What is the *purpose* of the U.S./Mexico border patrol?" If we look at the full name, "United States Customs and Border Protection" within the "Department of Homeland Security" we get the clear message that the purpose has more to do with "protection" of U.S. interests than attending to the sacredness of human life. If the function, purpose, or goal of this

entity was something more like the latter, a
more appropriate name may be something
like, "U.S. Customs and Border Safety" within
the "Department of Homeland Well-Being."

3. **Interconnections or Relationships**: According
to Meadows, this is the third highest leverage level
of intervention. *When you alter the nature of the
relationships (interconnections) in a system, you can
fundamentally shift the system.*

    a. For example, if border management and agents
were to undergo high quality relationship
building and communication training among
themselves, even aside from their interactions
with migrants, the outcomes of the border
patrol system would be significantly, perhaps
dramatically impacted. If you were to include
a global overhaul of border management
and agent relations with the people trying to
migrate across the border, you would alter the
system fundamentally.

4. **Elements**: This is where we start to lose steam in
terms of system leverage, and therefore, the potential
for real change. Unfortunately, many people don't
often look beyond this level. (When I say "beyond,"
as depicted in the image of this model, that means
"above.") When we look at human systems producing results we don't like, we often reflexively wonder,
"Who's in charge here?" mistakenly assuming that
replacing that person (which equates to replacing an

element in the system) will lead to "real change." As
Meadows says, a key person in a key position *can*
be the catalyst to alter an entire system. However,
this is the exception. More often, the "elements" (in
this case, people) in a system are ***highly replaceable***
(making that phrase italic, bold, and underlined on
purpose), and no matter who you replace, the system
will continue producing the same results it always
has. (That is, until someone or a group manages to
alter conditions at one of those earlier, higher up
levels.)

   a. In our example, changing *who* is in charge
      of border patrol, from local agents to chiefs
      to the president of the United States, you're
      likely to get the same system enacted again and
      again, despite your changes to leadership and
      personnel. Trump took the extreme approach
      of actually putting children in dog kennels.
      But his behavior was within the context of a
      long-standing system that would regularly put
      people in "holding cells" both before and after
      Trump.[8]

5. **Behavior**: If changing elements is low leverage,
   attempting to change behavior is even lower. Yet
   again, we often get fixated at this level, figuring that
   if we could just get "that person" or "them" to do

---

8   "Putting the U.S.-Mexico 'Border Crisis' Narrative into Context -
    Mexico," Relief Web, March 17, 2021, https://reliefweb.int/report/
    mexico/putting-us-mexico-border-crisis-narrative-context.

something other than what they are currently doing, then everything would be fine. It just doesn't work that way, and it's a waste of time to fixate here.

    a. This would look like providing training to border agents to alter their behavior. Unfortunately, these types of programs are often executed in the absence of in-depth conversations with the recipients of the "change program," failing to ask them what they think would be of benefit. Good change programs engender a higher level of insight, compassion, and communication or other skills needed for actors to make their own best decision in the moment. (But no matter how great the program, if the behavior of management stays the same then the change in the agents will be short-lived.)

6. **Events**: As Meadows says, this is "the nightly news," or the news headlines. Not only do we get fixated here, but the ever-streaming bad news haunts us, and sadly, negatively impacts our worldview (the top level of intervention). Attempting to change the world by focusing on events borders on madness. However, while it's not a strategy, in some cases it *is* a last resort.

    a. To return to our example, individuals with the group No More Deaths hike out into the desert and leave water and food for migrants, because unfortunately many migrants die of dehydration and starvation in the Arizona desert. During the Trump administration, border patrol was captured on video going out and destroying the water and food left for those migrants. It was later revealed that some of the footage was recent, and some not, and the activity was condemned by border patrol leadership. This back-and-forth at the level of events is the "madness" level where meaningful, sustainable change is, essentially, impossible.

To tie these two models together, consider that this last level, #6 Events, corresponds with the "Charitable / Direct Intervention" layer of the cake model above. In other words, we tend to direct our philanthropic dollars towards stopping bleeding, rather than upstream of the bleeding, towards the conditions that lead to suffering down the line.

Stepping Toward Change

Now that we have put these two models in place here are some recommended approximate steps towards achieving the SDGs in Marin. This is a set of basic ideas that are derived from and informed by Theory U, Collective Impact, and the Omidyar Group's "Systems Practice," in addition to the frameworks above. What I offer below contains key aspects that should not be overlooked, but neither should it be considered *the* roadmap. A key step is seeking out examples from other communities domestically or internationally where the locals have made sustained improvements in an issue area. But you must keep in mind that in complex, living systems, you can never lift a practice wholesale and simply paint it on to an entirely different community and expect it to work.

Step 0.0: The Agreement
This step consists of a general, community-wide agreement to adopt and adapt the SDGs. In this step, all municipalities in Marin, and the County of Marin publicly commit to meeting the UN Sustainable Development Goals by 2030, or on a timetable that makes sense within the local context, depending on the Goal or target.

Without city and county buy-in the effort is likely to remain limited to the same groups that have always done the heavy lifting: the local NGOs and community members doing their best, with government agencies and funders in the background doing business as usual, acting in isolation. Residents remain largely under-informed on all of these topics, with the important exception of small, private interests who voice their opposition in the line of NIMBYism (Not In My Back Yard). Residents *are* "Marin County," so we have to find a way for us to collectively take on this responsibility. (Note that many employees of local government and NGOs can't afford to live here, though many would like to. Naturally this impacts their level of investment in Marin. One can reasonably assume that it is hard to sincerely invest your whole self in a community that excludes you due to the cost of residential housing.)

Business tends to get involved at the charitable level. Only occasionally do they get involved at the level of advocacy.

However, their active support is most crucial at the level of systems, where the product or service they provide could shift from social and/or ecological liability to social and ecological benefit. (The wage floor at your business is a fundamental aspect of this.)

Steps 1 – 7: The Foundation

1. **Establish a backbone organization** for a given SDG following Collective Impact guidelines, with funding from individual donors, private and public foundations, the County, and local municipalities. (Note that in a small county such as Marin a single backbone may be appropriate for a collection of multiple SDGs; see step 5 below.)

2. **Establish communication norms** and commitment to those norms: Rely on organizational development and communication models (for example Nonviolent Communication, Powerful Non-Defensive Communication, Stretch Collaboration, etc.) to facilitate high quality communications in anticipation of inevitable disagreements and challenges. Earmark funds early on for professional support and training in this area. Your system is only as strong as your interconnections, so the more points of connection, and the stronger the connections, the better. Open communication and trust are the warp and woof of your system. The success of your efforts depends almost entirely on the quality of relationships in your system. Attending to

this is the first and most important job of leaders in the system.

3. **Qualify and define terms**: for example, what does Marin County mean by "poverty"? You want to hash out what various participants have in their head; make it verbal and write it down. But don't let this step drag out; it can take over and tank the process. As I learned from the Rise Together Leadership for Equity and Opportunity (LEO) trainings, "good enough" is often good enough. Rely heavily on definition of terms from outside organizations that specialize in this area, for example, look to PolicyLink for their "Equity Manifesto."

4. **Map the elements in the system** (which may be as simple as a table or list) in a way that is accessible and continually updatable by this particular group: "Who is already doing what?" Meadows notes that you often only need to map about 20% of a given system to get a working model. Don't get bogged down in trying to create an exhaustive map of a system that is constantly changing anyway. And don't expect complex maps created by outside entities to work for your group: mapping is meant to be done by the people doing the work; it will be imperfect and messy and will need to be updated and re-created on a rolling basis. Include NGOs, federal, state, and local government programs, school-based programs, businesses, and if possible, anecdotal information about strategies undertaken by private individuals

who are trying to make a difference in this issue
area. (See SDGMarin.org for a start on the list.)
Including free-agent community organizers and
community organizations (that are not necessarily
NGOs) is crucial.

5. **Map the interconnections in the system**: SDG #1
    "No Poverty" clearly overlaps with SDG #2 "Zero
    Hunger," and several others. The same upstream
    factors that lead to (downstream) homelessness also
    lead to (downstream) climate change (hence the
    Just Transitions movement). In a large social system,
    individual backbone organizations for every SDG
    makes sense, but their work will never bear fruit if
    they continue to work in isolated issue areas. In a
    smaller community like Marin, individual SDG
    groups may or may not make sense. In any case,
    interconnections should be attended to. For exam-
    ple, how does #3 "Good Health and Well-Being"
    overlap with #13 "Climate Action"? Where do #5
    "Gender Equality" and #15 "Life on Land" inter-
    sect? What opportunities are there to coordinate
    with those SDG groups to move toward positive
    change?

6. **Take stock**: Now that we have defined what we
    mean by X, we know where we want to get to *gen-
    erally* speaking, *and* we know who is already doing
    what, we can more carefully define local targets, and
    the boundaries of the system we want to significantly
    influence. Take stock of the picture as it has emerged

and ensure all stakeholders involved in the change process are fully informed before moving on to the next steps.

7. **Catalogue currently available measures**: How are these various organizations (and individuals if applicable) officially and unofficially defining and measuring progress? For example, for SDG #8 "Decent Work and Economic Development," you would want to reference the 2015 Comprehensive Economic Development Strategy (CEDS) from the Marin Economic Forum. For SDG #15 "Life on Land" you would want to reference the 2018 Rodenticide study, *Secondary Anticoagulant Rodenticide Exposure in Migrating Juvenile Red-Tailed Hawks in Relationship to Body Condition.* For human-focused SDGs, in addition to census data, what reports are available? In short, what is already available to illustrate our current state in relation to our goal?

Steps 8 – 10: Planning

8. **Engage the "Transformative Scenario Planning" process.** Use this method to clarify the current situation in relationship to a desired future, and specifically to clarify what the desired future looks like. Identify known, ongoing measures (for example, census data, Social Determinants of Health, Race Counts) to *define local targets under this Global Goal.* (For example, while Marin County doesn't have "extreme poverty," what do we want to see in Marin

by 2030 with regard to SDG #1 No Poverty?) Look for gaps; what is locally relevant that these already available indicators do not capture? Local targets may consist of wholesale adopting of Global Goal targets as published by the UN, slightly revising the text of existing global targets, and/or writing entirely new ones (that at least meet the global targets). First, draft targets, and second, define your terms.

9. **Approximate and establish** the financial and other resources necessary to meet these goals and targets. Easier said than done. Nevertheless, when you can demonstrate a clear need and a clear path toward closing a gap, you have a compelling narrative to present to potential supporters, from volunteers to donors to political actors.

10. **Clarify Responsibilities, Roles, and Timelines.** Now you have done the homework and the planning and you're ready for action. Step 10 is here to trigger the cyclical nature of this work. As the landscape shifts, things will continuously change. How are your efforts shaping up several months in? Is the future looking bright or grim already?

Step 11 - 12: Do & Review

11. This is the official **action step**, but in reality, action steps have already been taken all along the chain. Further, revisiting every step is necessary at some point; some are necessary to revisit on a regular basis.

12. **Review.** How is it going? The reason our most well-meaning NGOs and community group activities are not minting the results we want is in part due to our inability or unwillingness to honestly engage this step of honest review. (Another big missing piece is attending to the *purpose* question.) Did your backbone organization fall apart, or never really constitute in the first place? Did your top funder abandon you? Are people signing up to help and then disappearing? Don't despair! These problems are not going away, and in fact, are likely getting worse, so you have plenty of time to work on them. And even when you ameliorate a situation today, tomorrow brings new challenges.

    I'm only partially joking here. Living systems are always changing, and breaking out of our habit of expecting to "fix" anything is crucial to making the world a better place. We want to do our best today, *and* expect that tomorrow's people will both do better and have better ideas than we ever did. What can we do today to set them up to be better, smarter, more compassionate and capable that we are?

— CHAPTER 1 —

SDG #1 No Poverty

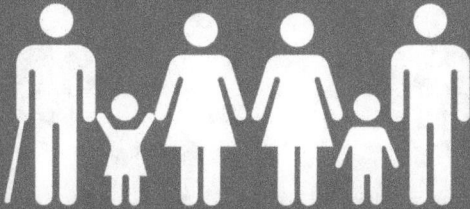

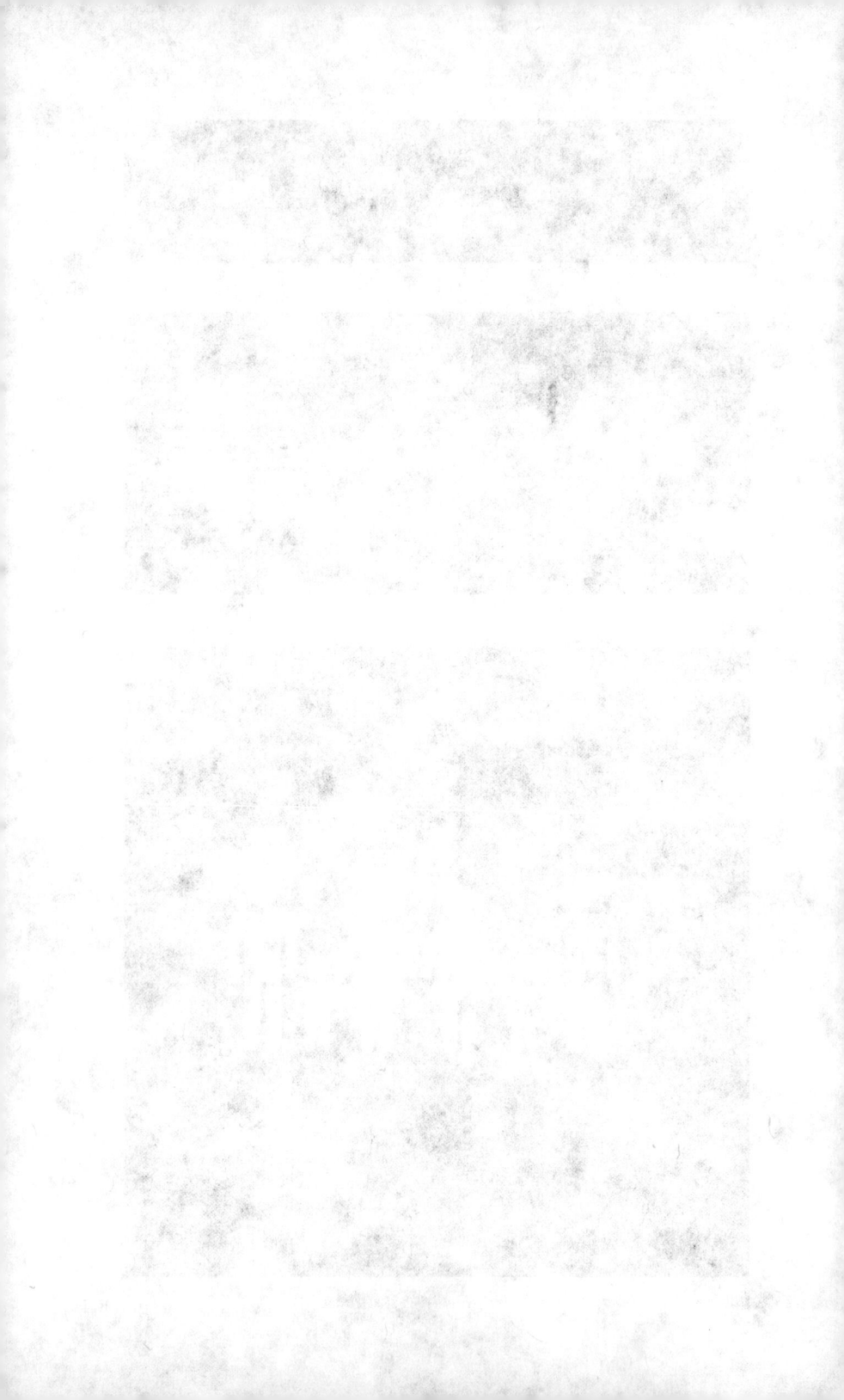

There are people who don't have a place to live!
We need to keep that in the forefront.

—ELBERTA ERIKSSON

Where Are We?

Rommel Carrera is originally from Ecuador. He worked for UNICEF (the United Nations Children's Fund, originally the United Nations International Children's Emergency Fund) in his home country, helping to build schools and create community development programs for the poor.

When moving to Marin County in 2016 he quickly recognized that what we call "poverty" here would be middle-class back in Ecuador. However, through his work he also saw that there is a certain relative quality to poverty, and those who live in poverty in Marin County do, indeed, suffer nearly insurmountable obstacles to entering the Marin middle class.

Families are living paycheck to paycheck, dealing with financial stress on a regular basis, trying to maintain a tenuous position in society. If you ask the people at First 5 Marin (our local Children and Families Commission, an independent government agency), this is even true about "middle class" families in Marin. For a family of four, if their combined household income is less than about $100,000, covering basic monthly expenses is a stretch, the major expenses being housing and childcare, not to mention medical expenses or other unexpected costs that can sink a family into debt that is nearly impossible to escape.

Does it make sense that families have to earn something approaching $150,000 annually just to be reasonably comfortable? Is that the world we want, or the world we want our kids to be faced with?

Native North Americans & the Challenges of Race-Based Reporting

Each chapter references limited statistics for American Indians or "Native North American" groups. Due to the nuances of statistics and vicissitudes of what individuals conducting studies choose to include or exclude, Native North Americans are usually left out of reports, and therefore don't appear in articles that discuss those reports and datasets.

Perhaps the main challenge is that there are so few Native North Americans compared to conventional racial groupings. Therefore, statisticians and researchers either overlook them or are forced to leave them out due to privacy concerns.

For example, if you are reporting graduation rates in a school district with 100 kids, 70% of whom are White, anything you say about that group is not easily traceable to any individual. Conversely, if there are only two Native North American kids in the group and you report the graduation rates of that ethnic group, everyone knows who you are talking about. This is the same as with any other very small minority group, and for all kinds of data.

Note that this is also true with regard to other groups that are of a relatively small size. For example, in this 88-page report from the U.S. Census Bureau, *Income and Poverty in the United States: 2019*, the only racial groups reported separately are White (with a "White, non-Hispanic" sub-group), Black, Asian, and Hispanic (any race). Footnotes state the following: "Data for American Indians and Alaska Natives, Native Hawaiians and Other Pacific Islanders, and those reporting two or more races are not shown separately".[9] They precede this statement in the footnotes with further explanation about racial categories, including, "The use of the single-race population does not imply that it is the preferred method of presenting or analyzing data."

One gets the feeling that it's all a little bit tortured, this endeavor of categorizing and counting people. Yet, it's the only way we currently have to understand when a particular group is excelling, keeping up, or falling behind in all number of measures of well-being.

Native Californians

If you have an interest in learning about the history of people native to what is now called "California," I highly recommend *Tending the Wild*, by M. Kat Anderson. (Anyone who owns property in California should have this book in their hands.) The 2020 census counted 9.7 million people who at least partially identify as American Indian or Alaska Native,[10] or

---

9   Jessica Semega et al., "Income and Poverty in the United States: 2019" (U.S. Department of Commerce, September 2020).

10 Rezal Adriana, "The States Where the Most Native Americans Live," US News, November 26, 2021, https://www.usnews.com/news/ best-states/articles/the-states-where-the-most-native-americans-live.

2.9% of the total American population at that time. California specifically has the second largest total number of individuals reporting Native American racial identity.[11]

How Did We Get Here?

This chapter for SDG #1 No Poverty includes the following additional framing to set the stage for the SDGs that follow.

Success to the Successful

There is a systems thinking concept called "success to the successful." You can learn more about it in Donella Meadow's book *Thinking in Systems: A Primer.* Essentially, it means that if you are winning today (i.e., wealthier), you're in a better position than those who are *not* winning today to keep winning over and above them tomorrow.

> *Using accumulated wealth, privilege, special access, or inside information to create more wealth, privilege, access or information are examples of the archetype called "successful to the successful."[. . .] That's a reinforcing feedback loop, which rapidly divides a system into winners who go on winning, and losers who go on losing.[12]*

---

11   "California Has the #2 Largest Native American Population in the U.S.," Stacker, November 22, 2021, https://stacker.com/california/california-has-2-largest-native-american-population-us.
12   Donella Meadows, *Thinking in Systems: A Primer* (Chelsea Green Publishing, 2008), 127.

This causes an inevitable stratification in the social system of which you are a part, and ultimately, the system breaks. (Many traditional societies have system controls in place to avoid social collapse, such as Jubilee year in Hebrew traditions, when all debts are forgiven, etc.) Unfortunately, as noted earlier, the increasing income gap between the poor and the wealthy demonstrates this systems trap in action.

One specific, local example is what is called "restrictive covenants" in property deeds. In plain language, this is language in your property deed that specifically states that the property cannot be sold to non-White people. Yes, this is illegal these days, but if you own property in Marin, depending on how old your title document is, it's possible this language exists in your property deed. The County of Marin put out a press release on October 27, 2022 stating the following:

Anyone living in a home built in the mid-1960s or earlier can examine their title papers and email the Recorder's Office staff if the racist restrictive covenants are found.[13]

Consider that it was the more successful group—White people—who were in a position to explicitly exclude non-Whites. We won't examine the details of accumulation of family wealth in relation to private property ownership, but you can infer the success to the successful phenomena in this example.

---

13 "County of Marin - News Releases - Restrictive Covenant Project," County of Marin, October 27, 2022, https://www.marincounty.org/main/county-press-releases/press-releases/2022/arcc-restrictive-covenants-102722.

Zooming back out again, success to the successful system trap is a *global* trend, so *local* action to reverse the trend must necessarily be extraordinarily robust to overcome the momentum of the global trend.

As you may imagine, this dynamic applies whether we're talking about SDG #1 No Poverty, #2 Zero Hunger, or any of the other social equity-related SDGs. (It also applies to the ecological SDGs, but less obviously.)

Federal Poverty Line

If I mention "poverty" to you as a Marin County resident, aside from extreme poverty as discussed above, you may reflexively refer to the federal poverty line. The federal poverty line is, as it turns out, extremely general, telling us very little of what we need to know about how people in our community are actually doing, financially or otherwise.

The Insight Center for Community Economic Development calls the federal poverty measure "antiquated".[14] Authors of a 2010 *Stanford Social Innovation Review* article explain that it is based solely on the cost of food, as opposed to taking into account the costs of other basics such as housing, transportation, and variations in the cost of living in your particular community.[15] A 2020 article on

---

14   "The Cost of Being Californian: A Look at the Economic Health of California Families," Insight Center, April 20, 2018, https://insightcced.org/2018-self-sufficiency-standard-report/.

15   Rourke O'Brien and David Pedulla, "Beyond the Poverty Line," Stanford Social Innovation Review, 2010, https://ssir.org/articles/entry/beyond_the_poverty_line.

americanprogress.org indicates that this situation has not improved in recent years:

> *If the United States hopes to end poverty, it needs to do a much better job of measuring it. That means creating official calculations that at least consider the real costs households face, that reflect mainstream standards of living, and that stay accurate over time. Failure to do so could have far-reaching consequences for decades to come.*[16]

California has one of the highest poverty rates in the country,[17] and inequality continues to grow. As noted above, this should signal to us that our efforts to reduce poverty in Marin will have to be particularly robust in that our work will be going against the tide of the state, and the nation.[18]

As of 2016, 7.2% of individuals who live in Marin County live at or below the federal poverty line,[19] or less than 19,000 of around 260,000 people. Note that these individuals are

---

16 Areeba Haider and Justin Schweitzer, "The Poverty Line Matters, but It Isn't Capturing Everyone It Should," Center for American Progress, March 5, 2020, https://www.americanprogress.org/article/poverty-line-matters-isnt-capturing-everyone/

17 Morgan Keith, "California Has the Highest Poverty Level of All States in the Us, According to Us Census Bureau Data," Business Insider, September 15, 2021, https://www.businessinsider.com/california-has-highest-poverty-level-in-the-us-census-bureau-2021-9.

18 Manuel Pastor, Vanessa Carter, and Jennifer Ito, "The Next California | Othering & Belonging Institute," Othering & Belonging Institute, April 18, 2018, https://belonging.berkeley.edu/next-california.

19 "People Living Below 100% of Federal Poverty Level, County: Marin," Healthy Marin, 2016, https://www.healthymarin.org/indicators/index/view?indicatorId=347&localeId=258.

considered to be living in poverty if their income is at or below
$12,880 (in 2021), or if the household income for a family of
four is at or below $26,500.[20]

Imagine trying to support yourself on $12,880 per year
($1,000 a month), the federal poverty cutoff line for a single
person. You would either be homeless, sleeping on someone's
couch, or if you were fortunate enough to have stable housing, heavily reliant on social programs (or the good graces
of friends and family) for your most basic necessities such as
food, medical care, and transportation.

Insufficient Minimum Wage
Wouldn't it be great if minimum wage jobs were at least
enough for a person to get by on? If that were the case, there
would be no difference between full-time employment and
what has been called "self-sufficiency." Unfortunately, due to
the fact that the minimum wage has 31% less buying power
than it did in 1968,[21] that is decidedly not the case. (You may
have heard of the "working poor" phenomenon.)

If you work a full-time minimum wage job, your take-home
pay is something like $1,600-$1,800 per month. You are

---

20 "U.S. Federal Poverty Guidelines Used to Determine Financial
    Eligibility for Certain Programs: HHS Poverty Guidelines for
    2022," Assistant Secretary for Planning and Evaluation, January 12,
    2022, https://aspe.hhs.gov/topics/poverty-economic-mobility/
    poverty-guidelines.
21 David Cooper, "Congress Has Never Let the Federal Minimum Wage
    Erode for This Long," Economic Policy Institute, accessed August 25,
    2022, https://www.epi.org/publication/congress-has-never-let-the-
    federal-minimum-wage-erode-for-this-long/.

unlikely to find *any* type of housing for less than $1,000 per month in Marin County. The $600 - $800 remainder *might* be enough to cover food, but not enough to cover transportation and household and personal care products, not to mention medical care and pharmaceuticals, or savings, and clothing for work and a haircut once in a while.

Are you thinking to yourself, "Well, what about Medicare? What about food stamps?" etc., then you have fallen into the trap of off-loading the cost of just basic survival from the employer to the government. In effect, taxpayers subsidize employers (and thereby, a perverse economic system) by providing these basic social services, enabling those employers to continue to pay unconscionably low wages. (Note that I'm suggesting here that the minimum wage should be reasonable, not that basic social services should *not* be provided.)

Self-Sufficiency Line

Instead, we have people working multiple jobs—sometimes multiple full-time jobs—but who are on the verge of losing their car, losing their home, or having to choose between medical care and paying a utility bill. This includes mothers who are unable to work even when they would like to because they can't afford to pay childcare; elders who are forced to continue working well past reasonable limits; young people who would like to live on their own but face having to leave their families behind and move to a more affordable area.

First 5 Marin has calculated that a family of four must have a total monthly income of $8,424, or $101,944 annually, to make ends meet. They have calculated that nearly one-quarter (23.1%) of families in Marin live below the self- sufficiency line.[22]

Marin Families - Self Sufficiency

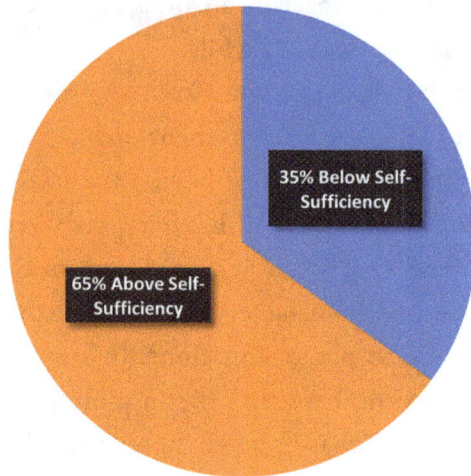

35% Below Self-Sufficiency

65% Above Self-Sufficiency

Figure 4 - Marin Residents, Self Sufficiency Line

The two most costly household expenses included in their calculation are housing, at $2,006, and childcare at $2,508 (plus food $758, transportation $397, healthcare $442, miscellaneous $618, taxes $1,962, and deductions for childcare tax credits -$267).[23]

---

22   "Self Sufficiency in Marin County," First 5 Marin, accessed August 25, 2022, https://www.first5marin.org/children-families-first/data-info/fact-sheets/self-sufficiency-in-marin-county/.

23   "Facing the High Cost of Living in Marin," First 5 Marin, accessed August 28, 2022, https://www.first5marin.org/children-families-first/data-info/fact-sheets/facing-the-high-cost-of-living-in-marin/.

There is a big gap between the federal poverty line and the self-sufficiency line. For a family/household of four people:

- Poverty $26,200 (Federal)[24]
- Self-Sufficiency (First 5 Marin) $101,944

The difference? $75,744. This dramatic gap underscores the profound inadequacy of the federal poverty line measure.

So Where Are We Really?

With these details in place, let's go back to the basic Global Goal: "End poverty in all its forms everywhere." The first target under this Global Goal, "By 2030, eradicate extreme poverty for all people everywhere, currently measured as people living on less than $1.25 a day," is nearly meaningless for many places in the world. Earning $456.25 per year in Marin County falls in this category. The next target is applicable to Marin County:

1.2 By 2030, reduce at least by half the proportion of men, women and children of all ages living in poverty in all its dimensions according to national definitions.[25]

24 "U.S. Federal Poverty Guidelines Used to Determine Financial Eligibility for Certain Programs: HHS Poverty Guidelines for 2022."
25 "Goal 1: End Poverty in All Its Forms Everywhere," United Nations Sustainable Development, accessed August 25, 2022, https://www.un.org/sustainabledevelopment/poverty/.

As discussed above, our national definition is the federal poverty line, which is $12,880 for an individual. If 7.2% of individuals in Marin County are currently at or below this line, we appear to be pretty close to meeting this Global Goal.

Marin Residents at or Below Federal Poverty Line

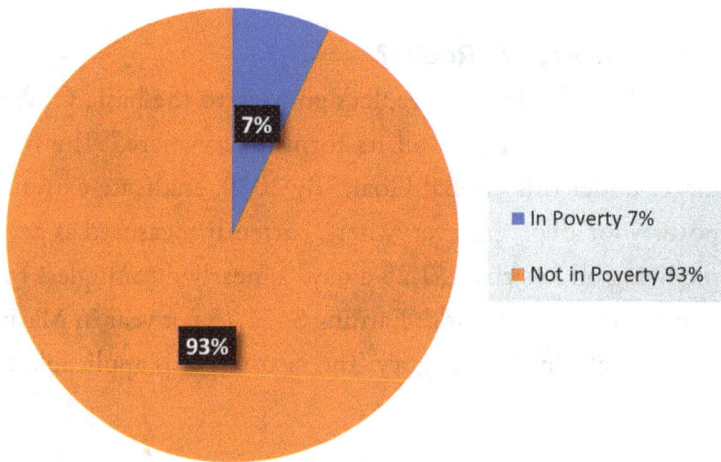

Figure 5 - Marin Residents, Federal Poverty Line, 2016

Note that this pie chart changes dramatically when we break it down by race, age, neighborhood, or other factors. This is where we have to ask ourselves as a community, "Where do we want to get to and by when, and *what indicators and measures will help us to get there?*"

Donella Meadows, referenced above, notes that you need to be really thoughtful about the measure or indicator you choose, because a system will tend to wrap itself around that number, for better *and* for worse. (She references GDP/GNP as an illustration of the dangers.) We have already established that the federal poverty line has been heavily critiqued, and some simple calculations, such as those above, tell you that it is extremely limited.

For a more realistic picture of poverty in Marin, we need to at least reference the self-sufficiency line. If anyone making less than the self-sufficiency income level in Marin County was counted as "living in poverty" then the graph above would be closer to a quarter of the pie graph.

Me as An Example
As someone who lives below the income level of what is considered self-sufficient, I would suggest that there is a gap between my simple lifestyle and what can reasonably be considered "poverty." Yes, I am reliant on publicly subsidized healthcare, but the healthcare system is so warped in favor of profit for the few that it skews everything. Yes, I live in an unconventional dwelling, but it is clean, relatively comfortable, affordable, and safe. Yes, I share a vehicle and associated costs with another person, but we both work from home so it kind of works out just fine. When I was unemployed and living on my friend's couch in Sausalito (for eight months. . . thank goodness for gracious friends), I would have been a much more likely candidate for the poverty category.

So if the federal poverty line is too low and the self-sufficiency standard may not accurately define what we tend to associate with "poverty" per se, we will need to turn to others in our community with a depth of knowledge in this area—most particularly low and very low-income individuals and families—for insights as to where to draw the line, and for the purposes of deciding together where we want to get to as a community.

Where Do We Want to Get to?

The Global Goal

The aspirational statement of this Sustainable Development Goal is, "End poverty, in all its forms, everywhere." That means no more poverty, period. As we have acknowledged, poverty in Marin County is of a less intense nature than poverty in the global South. At the same time, poverty here has real-world, negative consequences for individuals and society as a whole, across generations. And, at the state and national level it's getting worse. We have to ask ourselves, "What do we really want?" with regard to poverty in our county. Do we think it's ok for some people in Marin County to live in poverty? Or do we want to diminish all poverty "in all forms"? What, specifically, do we want to happen, and what, specifically, are we willing to do to reach those targets?

Global Targets Under SDG #1

Here is one example of a target under this Global Goal that could reasonably be adapted for Marin:

*1.4 By 2030, ensure that all men and women, in partic-
ular the poor and the vulnerable, have **equal rights to
economic resources**, as well as access to basic services, ownership and control over land and other forms of property,
inheritance, natural resources, appropriate new technology
and financial services, including microfinance [emphasis
added]*

Equal Rights to Economic Resources
Economic resources include things like access to bank
accounts, and credit and other loans at reasonable interest rates. This ties in with Global Goal #8 Decent Work &
Economic Growth. (Note that many activists replace the word
"Growth" with "Development" in SDG #8.) Perhaps the target
should say, "equal rights to *reasonable* economic resources," as
the poor are routinely made worse-off by financial institutions
such as banks and pay-day lending organizations. For example, this article, "Banking and Poverty: Why the Poor Turn to
Alternative Financial Services," describes the conditions that
lead to a downward spiral when low-income people take the
risk of joining the establishment, which wasn't designed for
them:

*Prepaid cards, check-cashing, and certain bank loans
appear, on the surface, to be the safe, convenient option
compared to alternative financial services that unbanked
and underbanked individuals heavily use. They are presented as a way to include the poor into banking systems.*

However, this inclusion comes at a hefty cost. [. . .] fees include purchase fees, monthly fees, ATM cash-withdrawal fees, ATM transaction-decline fees, balance inquiry fees, fees to receive a paper statement, dormancy fees, and many other fees that are not always disclosed.[26]

The text of the 1.4 target specifically names ". . . ownership and control over land and other forms of property. . . " This entails the option to purchase a home. But both income and race play big parts in denying this access; a topic that comes under the rubric of SDG #10: Reduced Inequalities (and SDG #11 Sustainable Cities and Communities). For example, a 2018 article claims, ". . . a new study found that African-Americans and Latinos were far more likely to be denied conventional mortgages than Whites, even when income, loan size and other factors were taken into account."[27] Another says, "The wealth gap between White and black Americans is widening: Black families now have 10 times less wealth than Whites."[28]

---

26 "Banking and Poverty: Why the Poor Turn to Alternative Financial Services," Berkeley Economic Review, accessed August 25, 2022, https://econreview.berkeley.edu/banking-and-poverty-why-the-poor-turn-to-alternative-financial-services/.

27 Emmanuel Martinez and Aaron Glantz, "For People of Color, Banks Are Shutting the Door to Homeownership," Reveal News, February 15, 2018, https://revealnews.org/article/for-people-of-color-banks-are-shutting-the-door-to-homeownership/.

28 Jennifer Streaks, "Black Families Have 10 Times Less Wealth than Whites and the Gap Is Widening—Here's Why," CNBC, 2018, https://www.cnbc.com/2018/05/18/credit-inequality-contributes-to-the-racial-wealth-gap.html.

Let's take another example target from this Global Goal:

1.5 By 2030, **build the resilience of the poor** *and those in vulnerable situations and reduce their exposure and vulnerability to climate-related extreme events and other economic, social and environmental shocks and disasters [emphasis added]*

Climate Resilience of the Poor

Continuing to look at equal rights and access issues, if you are at all familiar with the geography and neighborhoods of Marin County, you know that the Canal area of San Rafael is a largely Latino neighborhood, that Marin City has historically been an African American neighborhood, and that both are several feet from the bay waters. Marin City has a single entrance/exit route. These two neighborhoods are and will be among the first and hardest hit when it comes to stormwater surges. When faced with natural disasters, low-income families are the most vulnerable.

What might local targets for SDG #1 look like here?

My recommendation to Marin County, and really, any community that cares enough to engage with the Global Goals, is to set local targets. A cross-organization, cross-sector coalition would set local targets for meeting Global Goal #1 No Poverty in Marin County. The local targets need to spring from the hearts and minds of the people living in poverty and below the self-sufficiency threshold, and from the people who are already working to address the symptoms and causes of poverty in Marin.

Further, after attending dozens (and dozens) of community meetings in Marin County between 2017 and 2022, it's clear to me that meeting a high bar for positive change will require the buy-in and active participation of thousands of Marin County residents of all income levels; far more than the number currently involved. It is up to us to take active responsibility for the health and well-being of our own community. *We are Marin*; no one else is going to make this happen for us. (I have heard anecdotally from community organizers that they are challenged when seeking funding from sources from *outside* of Marin because potential funders say, "But you guys have the Marin Community Foundation; why would you need help from us?")

To start thinking about setting local targets under this SDG, let's take the second target under SDG #1:

1.2 By 2030, reduce at least by half the proportion of men, women and children of all ages living in poverty in all its dimensions according to national definitions.[29]

On its face this would mean for Marin something like the following:

Marin County will reduce by at least half the proportion of men, women and children of all ages living in poverty in all its dimensions according to the federal poverty line.

---

29   UNDP, "Goal 1 End Poverty in All Its Forms Everywhere."

We have already discussed the issues with the federal poverty line, so that aspect could and likely should be replaced. But for illustration purposes, here are some possibilities of what this might look like:

By December of 2030 no more than 3.8%, or less than 9,600 people in Marin County will live at or below the federal poverty line.

Perhaps something could be added to this target such as, "... as a result of well-being initiatives, not displacement." After all, simply pushing out even more poor people from Marin County would be one artificial way to meet this Goal. (But of course, this tactic would exacerbate factors for other Global Goals, not the least of which is #10 Reduced Inequalities, in addition to traffic under SDG #11 Sustainable Cities and Communities.)

The phrase "poverty in all its forms," however, implicates the self-sufficiency measure. A variation, or additional target, could be:

By December of 2030 no more than 12% of families in Marin County will live below the self-sufficiency line.

This would be a significant change from nearly 25% of families living below self-sufficiency today, as referenced earlier in this chapter.

How Do We Get There?

General ideas for next steps are supplied in the Introduction. Specific steps would flow from those, especially from a cross-section of people who already work in this area. However, most importantly, the actual direction must come from average, everyday Marin County residents who are directly or indirectly impacted by poverty and low-income living, either because they are a member of that group, have friends and loved ones who are, or who are simply concerned members of society.

(Note: We are not talking about yet another set of workshops gathering input from participants who fill up large sheets of paper followed by not-a-whole-lot. We're talking about putting infrastructure in place that facilitates the realization of that input, much of which has already been gathered in years past and is sitting in the closets of various community organizers and community organizations.)

The topics below are included as they strongly pertain to this SDG, and in some cases, the social equity topic more generally.

Upward or Social Mobility

It's not for everyone.
First, I want to acknowledge that not everyone wants to ascend the social ladder, and nor should they be expected to. We have a massive bias in this society toward ever-accumulating material wealth, and that's just not everyone's focus. Cultural, familial,

and life circumstances all influence whether a person is, for example, striving for their third car, or content to share one with others; working on attaining that elusive vacation home, or happily sharing a home with multiple generations of their family under one roof. Rather, the concern here is at least two-fold. Is a given individual able to maintain a reasonable level of health and well-being, or are they suffering due to constraints society is imposing? Are opportunities available for a person to live up to their full potential? Finally, when we add in the systems perspective, is that person able to fulfill their aspirations in a way that is socially and ecologically sustainable? Or do they feel they have to compromise their values to "get ahead"?

The Global Social Mobility Index
The Global Social Mobility Index of 2020—from the World Economic Forum—rated 82 countries on their "social mobility." This is a measure of a person's capacity to move up from the economic conditions of their parents. More accurately, it's a measure of a country's support for individuals to do so.

The report found that globally, "... most economies are failing to provide the conditions in which their citizens can thrive, often by a large margin".[30] The United States was not in the top five; not in the top ten; not in the top 20. We're number 27 in terms of upward social mobility. That means that despite the dominant narrative of the U.S. being the "land of opportunity," there are 26 other countries ahead of us in that regard.

---

30 "Global Social Mobility Index 2020," World Economic Forum, January 19, 2020, https://www.weforum.org/reports/global-social-mobility-index-2020-why-economies-benefit-from-fixing-inequality/.

Do we have a systems-level approach here in Marin?
Marin is much like most other places in that we do not have a systems-level approach to managing our society or making it a better, healthier, more prosperous place for people to live. What we do have are a number of charitable/direct service efforts (that top layer of the cake model covered in the Introduction) and a handful of advocacy organizations (the latter in particular with regard to the environment). Unfortunately, very few of our local advocacy organizations take an active, public stand in favor of greater economic equity.

There are many organizations and some local government agencies in Marin County that attend to individuals and families who need help in the face of utility bills they can't cover, emergency help with rent, clothing, food, and homelessness. Please take note: alleviating the *symptoms* of poverty is different from alleviating the *upstream causes* of poverty. So far, our society has not turned off the tap on factors that lead to people living in poverty. Rather, we make some effort to hold out a bucket and catch people before they go down the drain and end up in the proverbial gutter.

Some organizations do both when it comes to individuals. For example, Canal Alliance in San Rafael offers programs for immigrants in particular to continue their education, learn English, and learn job skills, while also offering immediate emergency help such as a food pantry, emergency rent and utility assistance, and emotional and behavioral health services. This is an example of trying to support individuals in their attempts to interface with the existing system in a way that allows them to be more successful within it.

With regard to the upstream causes of poverty in the system itself, organizations such as the group North Bay Jobs with Justice, based in Sonoma County, provide examples. This group in particular spearheaded the successful City of Novato minimum wage increase campaign, discussed below. This particular campaign targeted an important, fundamental upstream condition: local minimum wage. The Economic Security Project, which challenges mega-monopolies and advocates for initiatives such as universal basic income, is another example of going upstream to enact fundamental changes to the existing system.

So, what needs to change?

"Best Practices"

Contrary to popular belief, it is not and cannot be the job of nonprofit organizations to tackle the society-wide conditions that lead to poverty, though many try valiantly. Poverty versus prosperity is a huge complex of factors for which all of society is responsible. You are responsible. I am responsible. All local businesses have a role to play that is no less important than local NGOs or the government. Only through the "best practice" of cross-sector strategy, coordination, alignment and synergy can we successfully reverse the current, dominant trend. (Keep in mind that the term "best practices" is a bit of a trope. It can just as easily be an empty platitude as it can be a useful reference.)

Complexity

Clearly with the question of poverty we are in the realm of the complex, and systems thinking helps us to *hold* rather than artificially *reduce* complexity. Establishing the conditions necessary for everyone to have equal access to a prosperous, fulfilled life is not and won't be easy; the rest of the country dwarfs Marin County, and the behemoth is moving in the wrong direction. But also, we have a considerable amount of local control, and we have yet to maximize our engagement with those local opportunities. We need to hold both of these truths, to move into the complexity, rather than artificially reduce things down to linear plans that are ill equipped to successfully navigate complexity.

Here is one local example of people taking responsibility for the well-being of the lowest earners in their community.

City of Novato Minimum Wage
In 2019 the City of Novato took a step (unprecedented in Marin County, but happily, increasingly common throughout the Bay Area) and increased their local minimum wage. Having attended three public hearings on this matter I can tell you that the pushback was extreme, at times disturbing. (I spoke with one business owner who wanted to support the initiative, but who had been aggressively intimidated by other business owners in the past on another issue, so they didn't speak up this time.) In 2020 the same opponents pushed back again, citing COVID as the reason. To their credit, the Novato City Council held firm, recognizing the negative systemic impact an inadequate minimum wage has on their community, and the even greater need to support the most vulnerable in pandemic times.

What do we want instead? People working in local governments need to step outside the box. Residents (at *all* socioeconomic levels) must be at the heart of the process, as supporters, as subject matter experts, and as the most important "target market": those most invested in seeing their county fundamentally transform. Businesses have the opportunity to become strategic partners, ideally becoming co-ops and Benefit Corporations ("B Corps") where possible.

Do we have the collective will, in Marin, to come together to dramatically reduce or eliminate poverty *here*? If we do not, it's unlikely that outside forces will do this *for* Marin residents. Our society is becoming more stratified, with the middle class shrinking. According to Investopedia, "In 2021, just 50% of American adults lived in middle-income households—down from 54% in 2001, 59% in 1981, and 61% in 1971. The middle class has been both decreasing in population share and seeing its cut of the income pie shrink."[31] The shrinking of the middle class—as has been happening here in Marin for decades—should be an alarm bell. According to research, and perhaps common sense, it is the middle class—not the wealthy—who have the best shot at mental and emotional well-being.[32,33]

31   Jake Frankenfield, "What Is Middle Class Income? The Latest Numbers Available," Investopedia, July 14, 2022, https://www.investopedia.com/financial-edge/0912/which-income-class-are-you.aspx

32   Amy Patterson Neubert, "Money Only Buys Happiness for a Certain Amount," Purdue University, February 13, 2018, https://www.purdue.edu/newsroom/releases/2018/Q1/money-only-buys-happiness-for-a-certain-amount.html.

33   Audrey Hamilton and Suniya Luthar, "The Mental Price of Affluence," Speaking of Psychology, accessed December 1, 2022, https://www.apa.org/news/podcasts/speaking-of-psychology/affluence.

CHAPTER 2

SDG #2 Zero Hunger

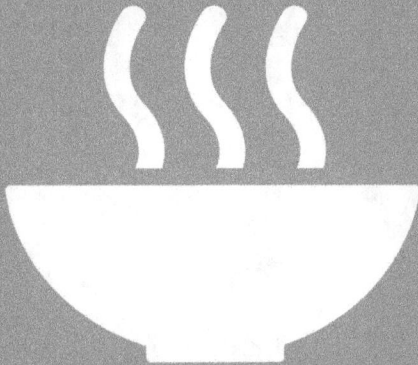

I remember quart jars out on the porch full
of something green. . . . and we were hungry
enough that I took those quart jars and I
dumped them into a pot and I boiled them, for
hours. I boiled them and then we ate it. Now if
that happens to you, you remember it.
—Pam Drew, Novato City Council meeting[34]

Where Are We?

"Food Stamps" & CalFresh

I grew up in Nevada County, which—despite the name—is in Northeastern California. In our really tiny, rural town, we were one of many families living at least in part on public assistance programs. Thus, doing some research recently, I experienced a time travel moment when I ran across images of what were called "food stamps" from the 1980s. I recognized those colored pieces of money-like paper from my childhood.

"Food stamps" are no longer in existence in the same form. The national program is now called Supplemental Nutrition Assistance Program (SNAP), and in California, this exact same program is branded as "CalFresh." (It was only when doing

---

34 "Joint City Council / City Council as Successor Agency Meeting," City of Novato, 2019. https://novato.granicus.com/player/clip/1521?view_id=7&redirect=true&h=181db227a6ee4e0c72165fe78b5c9bdb.

research for this book that I got these two terms straight.) CalFresh is the largest source of food assistance for individuals and families in California.

A friend said to me one day, "There are hungry people in Marin?" At first I was shocked. *How could you not know?!* I thought. But after a moment's reflection, I realized, *How* would *you know?* With the important exception of the Summer 2019 issue of *Edible Marin & Wine Country* magazine, titled "The Issue of Hunger," food access topics rarely make front page news in Marin.

The bulk of this chapter takes a fairly linear approach. Below I reference reports that document the gap between people and food, and how many people there are who lack reliable access to reasonable food.

However, when it comes to *doing something* about this issue, a linear approach is insufficient. Therefore, we'll discuss "food sovereignty" and "food sheds" in the later part of this chapter. (Note that the food system itself is made up of many workers who are themselves "food-insecure," including farmers in Marin County.)

If you find the following, more linear data coverage tedious, feel free to skip ahead to the "Where do we want to get to?" section of this chapter. Don't let the seeming mundane nature of food fool you: food is perhaps our biggest, most obvious access point to visioning and moving towards a truly inspiring, sustainable society, both locally and globally.

"Hunger"

Upon the mention of "hunger," people usually see images of far-off places with people literally dying on the side of the road or in desert huts. Marin County does not have this extreme level of hunger leading to wasting and death. What we face is the impact of **challenged access to nutritious, affordable food**, repeatedly, over time.

Due to income constraints and competing costs such as housing, medicine and healthcare, transportation, etc., the quality of food consumed by low and very low-income individuals is often compromised, to say the least. Further, people without kitchens or at least a refrigerator and a way to heat up food are even further limited; they either have to purchase prepared food (which is more expensive and/or less nutritious), receive prepared food for free, or survive on raw produce and packaged food.

This ongoing struggle is real and significant for a number of individuals and families in Marin. Food access-related duress impacts not just physical, but mental well-being, considering the stresses of trying to provide food for your family when there is not enough money to meet all immediate needs. The stress of the stigma related to receiving "handouts" is a significant added burden.

There is a gray area between "hunger" and food access challenges. I for one don't recall going hungry when I was a child, yet my parents—my mom in particular—were regularly stressed about money and food. As a low-income family, it seemed there was always some kind of scramble going on.

The quality of food, no matter the source, is another matter. Much of what passes for food today is *pseudo* food, more appropriately termed a "semi-edible industrial product."

As a child, I personally did not relish powdered milk, which we received in plastic bags from the food bank. But our 1980-something powdered milk was perhaps more nutritious than many of the packaged "foods" on the shelves of today's large grocery stores.

"Missing Meals"

The Missing Meals report is one way people who work on this issue have attempted to clarify how many individuals and families are food-insecure. According to the 2019 fact sheet about hunger in Marin, about 1 in 5 people in Marin County are "at risk of food insecurity." The Missing Meals Report has been compiled by various organizations over the past few years. The 2019 report and fact sheet was carried out by the San Francisco–Marin Food Bank.

I have to admit, I find this "missing meals" metric confusing. The report cites that "10.5 million meals are 'missing' in Marin County." I have a hard time conceptualizing how that translates to humans, which we will try to do in a moment. But first, I will explain how the authors of the report get to that number, and of course, I suggest refering to the original report for details.

The Numbers

I'm going to explain how they calculate missing meals, but if you don't quite follow, that's ok: I will provide a more general interpretation later.

First, they take the total number of people in Marin County (based on census data) living below 200% of the federal poverty line. That was 47,700 people in 2017 (which is about 6,000 people less than the population of Novato). Assuming each person in this group requires three meals per day, they then tally the *total* number of meals needed by this group in a year. That gave them 52 million meals.

What they are interested in is this: what is the gap? What is the gap between total meals one would reasonably expect this low-income group to consume, and the number of meals they could reasonably be expected to purchase or have access to via a service of some kind?

This is where it gets more complex, and they speak to this in the longer Missing Meals report. How do you know how much money a family allocates to food versus other necessities and expenses? You'll have to read the report for the longer explanation. Suffice it to say that aside from calculating the number of meals the family can reasonably be expected to purchase (again, based on their income level), one must also take into account meals that come from public assistance and charitable programs, like school lunches, CalFresh, food banks and pantries, and any other community support program that keeps records they are willing to share publicly.

Of the 52 million meals needed in total by 47,700 people in 2017, 10.5 million were said to be "missing." *That* is the gap.

Here's the general interpretation:

- In 2017, this group of 47,700 can be expected to afford 27 million of the 52 million meals needed.

- Another 9 million meals were provided by various government programs.
- An additional 6 million were provided by nonprofit organizations.
- That leaves a gap of 10.5 million meals "missing," or one in five (20%).

FYI, 10.5 million is an increase in missing meals by 23% from 2009, but it has hovered around the same level since about 2011.

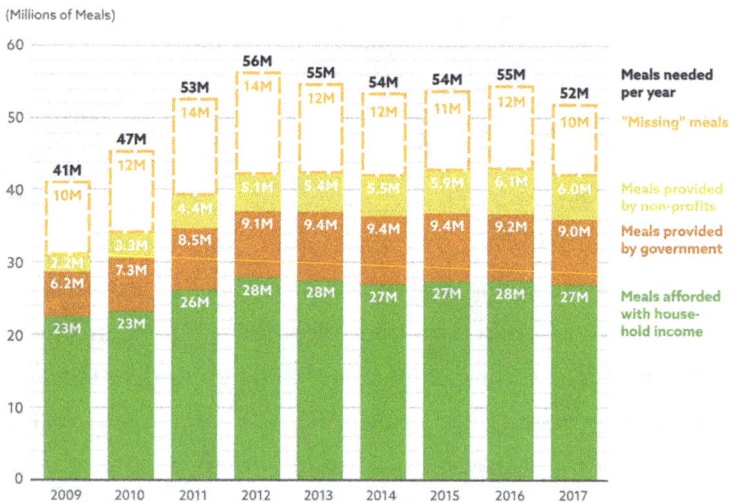

Figure 6 - "Missing Meals" in Marin, San Francisco-Marin Food Bank 2019 Fact Sheet

Additional Calculation Methods

Of course, if you're like me, you only loosely identify with this standardized approach to quantifying meals and food access. I don't have a better idea on how to measure food access issues, but there are other ways to look at this situation.

One way is to look at the number of people on CalFresh in Marin County. According to the CalFresh "tableau" dashboard, 5,265 households in Marin participated in CalFresh in 2019. (That number went up to 8,006 in 2020 with the pandemic.) Note this is *households* as opposed to individuals. According to the *Lost Dollars, Empty Plates* 2019 report from California Food Policy Advocates, an estimated 1.7 million Californians are eligible for CalFresh but not receiving benefits. They don't say what that gap is for Marin County specifically, however, the point of the report is the following: if everyone in California who is eligible for CalFresh enrolled, California would have received from the federal government an additional $1.8 billion in CalFresh dollars, which would have led to an additional $3.3 billion in economic activity. (For which year? It's an average derived from data for the federal fiscal years 2016 – 2019.[35])

Marin County's portion of this is: we would have received an additional $14,600,000 dollars to our county for this program, resulting in an additional $26,100,000 in economic activity.[36] Therefore, there is a positive economic benefit to local economies when all eligible individuals and families *do* use CalFresh. Local businesses receive additional revenue when people use their CalFresh benefits in their establishments.

---

35 "Lost Dollars, Empty Plates What CalFresh Means for Individuals & the Economy," California Food Policy Advocates, 2019, https://nourishca.org/CalFresh/CFPAPublications/LDEP-FullReport-2019.pdf.
36 Ibid., 4.

Another approach is to look at neighborhoods, and whether or not people have ready access to fresh produce and grocery stores within walking distance (considering many low-income people do not have ready access to reliable transportation). In recent years a large grocery store has moved into the Canal neighborhood of San Rafael, and Target—including some version of groceries—has moved into the Gateway Shopping Center in Marin City. While this is an improvement in both cases, interviews of local residents would need to be done to determine if this is sufficient to reasonably meet their needs.

Where do we want to get to?

In 2018, while attending a community meeting in Marin City, someone piped up, "If you don't own a home, you are home-less." As someone who has only ever rented since moving out of my dorm room in 1999, I have to say I could feel a certain confrontational truth in what he said.

If we turn that around to apply to food, we could say something like, "If you don't produce your own food you are food insecure." Or maybe, given that food production has histor-ically been communal, "If your community doesn't produce its own food, your community is food insecure." The idea of a "food shed" applies here, as in the geographic region in which the food is produced and consumed.[37]

---

37   Kristine Hahn, "What Is a Food Shed?," College of Agriculture and Natural Resources, March 24, 2013, https://www.canr.msu.edu/news/what_is_a_food_shed.

Food Sovereignty

Where do we want to get to? Answer: "food sovereignty," the definition of which provides an excellent answer to this question:

> *Food sovereignty is the right of peoples to healthy and culturally appropriate food produced through ecologically sound and sustainable methods, and their right to define their own food and agriculture systems. It puts the aspirations and needs of those who produce, distribute and consume food at the heart of food systems and policies rather than the demands of markets and corporations.*
> *– Declaration of Nyéléni, the first global forum on food sovereignty, Mali, 2007.[38]*

In the age of agribusiness, food production has become industrial, and global. It is entirely dependent on fossil fuel. Disruption in fossil fuel supplies have impacts on global food supplies. From making tools, to running planting, harvesting, and processing machinery, to transportation and all distribution, fossil fuels make this global network of food production and distribution possible.

We in Marin County are not at all insulated from this reality. We are as much a part of this globalized food system as any other county in the Bay Area.

---

38   "Food Sovereignty," US Food Sovereignty Alliance, 2007, http:// usfoodsovereigntyalliance.org/what-is-food-sovereignty/.

Before we get to more details of a vision, let's review some of the SDG targets.

SDG #2 Targets

Of the five main SDG #2 global targets, all five have some aspects that could be reasonably interpreted to fit our local context. Here is the first target under SDG #2:

2.1 By 2030, end hunger and ensure access by all people, in particular the poor and people in vulnerable situations, including infants, to safe, nutritious and sufficient food all year round.

What would this look like in Marin?

We will discuss that in a moment. First, however, I'd like to make the strong suggestion that we set the bar considerably higher than this target suggests.

The Vision

Here I suggest three levels of magnitude in terms of potential change.

Sustainable

It is tempting to call this the "Highest Vision" or to label it "The Ideal." But in reality, it's the only literally "sustainable" version of a food system of the three versions I lay out here. A truly sustainable vision also needs to be inspirational, like the food sovereignty statement.

In this visionary scenario the "missing meals" report has become totally irrelevant, because there is such a high level of local, sustainable food production (as in permaculture) for both personal and collective consumption that we are looking to help neighboring counties because we have such abundance. *Everyone* grows *something*, whether in their yard, on their patio or balcony, rooftop, or a community garden plot. Food and the food system have moved from a basic necessity (that occasionally becomes more interesting only in fancy fundraisers or restaurant contexts) to a vibrant system about which everyone is fairly well informed and active within. In short, it's a substantial culture change around food.

We have achieved food sovereignty and are well positioned to survive the ecological and economic storms of climate change and other major disruptions.

Interim

We've moved from a tiny percentage of locally-grown food being consumed locally to something more like 40 percent. (What precisely qualifies as "local" would have to be determined.) Gone are the days of "No chickens allowed in this neighborhood," or "This HOA won't let you have a vegetable garden in your front yard," or neighbors complaining that your citrus tree is (gasp) reaching into their yard. (Note that if we're going to eat meat locally this also means at least one local slaughterhouse.) Permaculture is known and embraced by most food growers. Food system employees no longer have to work multiple full-time jobs; they are paid well enough that they no longer routinely qualify for public food assistance.

Lowest Hanging Fruit

This is current business as usual, incrementally improved. The Marin Food Policy Council (see the section about them below) gets improved, sustainable funding, and SDG #2 becomes common knowledge. Zoning and other policy that obstructs local food production are chipped away at. There is a higher level of coordination across producers in terms of the waste-equals-food network. There is also a higher level of coordination between producers, processors, distributors, and consumers such that less is wasted, food-miles-traveled are reduced, and wages are improved.

Would we be happy with closing the "missing meals" gap? Is that where we want to get to? Or do we want a food system in which the workers in that system are able to reliably afford their own (damn) food? Maybe we want to aim for something socially and ecologically sustainable, like a food system that works for 100% of people 100% of the time, even in the face of disasters?

How do we get there?

According to an article on the NPR website, "Your Grandparents Spent More Of Their Money On Food Than You Do," Americans in 1960 spent 17.5% of their household income on food[39]. As of 2013, that was closer to 10%. This

---

39   Eliza Barclay, "Your Grandparents Spent More Of Their Money On Food Than You Do," NPR.org, March 2, 2015, https://www.npr.org/sections/thesalt/2015/03/02/389578089/your-grandparents-spent-more-of-their-money-on-food-than-you-do.

drop represents many factors, from falling food prices (and, unfortunately, falling quality) to rising housing, medical, and other household costs. This change is indicative of a system that has undergone massive shifts over recent decades. Food production and distribution has become increasingly global, and increasingly homogenized. In short, it has become less about feeding people and supporting small farmers and more about profit and agribusiness. If you think that should lead us to ask about the "purpose" of the food production system in this country, then you are on the right track.

The Marin Food Policy Council (MFPC)

In 2017, I began attending the monthly meetings of the Marin Food Policy Council. If that name is confusing—as it was to me for the first year—just take the word "policy" out of it and you'll get the gist. It's made up by a group of people from local government and nonprofits who get together once a month (about 95% women) to try to improve their efforts to address food access issues across Marin. This often means signing on to support or oppose legislation at the local, state, and federal level. The legislation policies discussed help or hinder the ability of residents to readily access nutritious, sustainable, affordable food. (A typical example might be allocation of state funding that impacts school lunch availability.)

Attending my first MFPC meeting, I was happy to discover that they had the benefit of a couple of quarter-time paid staff from the local U.C. Davis Agricultural Extension (another confusing title) and were remarkably organized, dutifully taking minutes they later publish, and following Robert's Rules

of Order. (MFPC's meetings are public so feel free to attend.)
Soon I sniffed out their systems thinking roots, discovering
that their founders were ecoliteracy people. ("Ecoliteracy" is a
systems thinking framework from Fritjof Capra that promotes
what it sounds like, "ecological literacy," as a way primarily for
students to develop a systems view of our world.)

The Potential

The Marin Food Policy Council has the potential to be
the backbone organizer for closing the gap between food
and people in Marin County. Participants are heavily tilted
toward professionals in the NGO and local government sectors. Local farmers, interested residents, and people who currently (or in the past) suffer from food insecurity are largely
missing. But the organized, focused structure and spirit of
the Council, along with its longevity, position it to be a great
platform for a much more robust effort to coordinate food
security work.

Healthy Eating Active Living (HEAL) Initiative

This is another local body well positioned to take on the backbone role of #2 Zero Hunger. I only learned about HEAL
about a year into my time attending Marin Food Policy
Council meetings, which tells me that if the Council is largely
a place for local government and NGO insiders to address
food access, the HEAL initiative is even more so.

Nevertheless, I heard a rumor that the stated goal of HEAL
is to end hunger in Marin County. As of this writing I am
unable to find anything on their website that clearly states this

as a goal for the initiative, much less a timeline and a plan, but if the group has landed on this as their mission, that's great news.

Agricultural Institute of Marin (AIM)

I don't know a whole lot about AIM, but it and organizations like it are of paramount importance to help us—as item #1 in their strategic plan says[40]—"Strengthen local and regional food systems." Going back to the "Where do we want to get to" portion of this chapter, one can say that very few people in Marin County are "food secure," in that very few people produce their own food. If, or rather, *when* catastrophe strikes food supply chains, our food intake will be interrupted. When your food shed is global and profit-driven, it is weak and subject to disruption from far and near. Moreover, those food supply chains depend on fossil fuel—the longer the path from farm to plate, the greater that dependence, and the larger the carbon footprint.

Organizations such as AIM are crucial to changing this reality. It's very questionable just what percentage of the food *eaten* locally can reasonably be *grown* locally, due to land and water constraints. However, we've not even begun to explore that question as far as I can tell, and I've been paying attention.

---

40 Agricultural Institute of Marin, "Agricultural Institute of Marin: 3-Year Strategic Plan, 2021 – 2024," January 2021, 5, https://static1. squarespace.com/static/5fd7b5e8b59b81291926f482/t/60124a7f-4769884fa732840b/1611811456710/Agricultural+Institute+of+M arin+3-+Year+Strategic+Plan+Final.pdf.

Next Steps

As with SDG #1 No Poverty, the role of the food system at large needs to be examined, and more specifically, the purpose of the larger system. As long as the dominant food system is run by organizations with profit as *the* goal, some people will be priced out of real food. Further, the profit motive tends to drive greater and greater homogenization of a given sector, that is, greater and greater consolidation of smaller outfits into ever-larger corporate entities. Small, more distributed food production is the key to greater food resilience throughout the system, and that includes Marin County.

The most important contributor to the local food system is and always has been the farmer, whether small or large scale. However, the larger, more automated and distant the farm, the more divorced the production is from the reality of the person consuming the food at the other end. Nutrition, wages, quality, ecological health. . . all are degraded in this gap.

With the help of some versions of the steps outlined in the Introduction to this book, Marin County can clarify just how food secure we are or are not, consider the size of our environmental impact due to food production, and sketch a potential path toward food sovereignty. This is a leap beyond "food security" to a paradigm (to use a 50-cent word) in which the people who produce the food are leaders and full participants in the decision-making processes that go into food system stewarding. (An important aspect is also culturally appropriate food.)

Food is potent. As you can see, it overlaps with many other issue areas, so we will see it pop up again and again in the remainder of this book. It could be the main entry point for organizing a socially just, ecologically sustainable society.

CHAPTER 3

SDG #3 Good Health and Well-Being

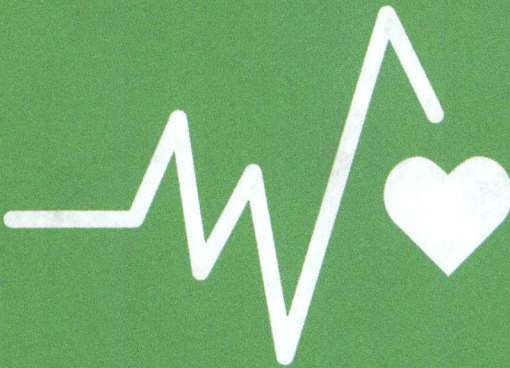

Where are we?

I nitially, I thought that this chapter would be fairly straight-forward to write. Of all the SDGs, data on health is readily available. Further, Marin is "pretty healthy" already. However, I struggled to really get into this chapter and make it work. Here's why.

Yes, data is readily available. You may have heard anecdotally that Marin County is "the healthiest county in California." This is according to the *County Health Rankings & Roadmap* report, which is published annually for the entire United States. This report looks at a great variety of statistics, from smoking and alcohol use to mental health days taken, to the usual instances of disease per 100,000 people, age at death, infant mortality rates, car accident injuries and deaths, and so on.

Health statistics also provide top examples of what are referred to as "disparities," meaning, some groups do really well, and others really not well, largely along economic lines, as well as race. (You may have heard anecdotally that "health and wealth" go together.) Marin's large group of doing-really-well hides the small pockets of Marin communities that have lower than average health. More on that later.

But the underlying issue that took a while to bubble up is the fact that our current "health" system is, as many have observed, more of a "sick" system. It is almost entirely reactionary and is decidedly mechanistic: the antithesis of a systems approach.

That is precisely what tripped me up when attempting to draft this chapter.

How do we know that what we have is actually more of a sick system? As Hilary Cottam observes in *Radical Help*, discussing the National Health Service (NHS) in the UK, "The NHS is founded on an idea that it can cure: it can administer a pill or an operation and we will be well. This model is well honed and still important – we need hip replacements, antibiotics and emergency procedures – **but it doesn't work for chronic problems.**"[41]

The U.S. has a similar (perhaps identical) worldview to the UK when it comes to healthcare—or sick care. It can respond to punctual emergencies. But it limps along when it comes to the epidemic of chronic disease.

Fritjof Capra and Pier Luigi Luisi in *The Systems View of Life: A Unifying Vision,* a systems thinking textbook, explain this mechanistic versus systemic approach to healthcare:

> *Rather than asking why an illness occurs and trying to remove the conditions that lead to it, medical researchers and practitioners often limit themselves to understanding the mechanism through which the disease operates, so that they can then interfere with them.*
>
> *A systemic approach, by contrast, would broaden the scope from the level of organs and cells to the whole person ... Although every practicing physician knows that healing is*

---

41   Hilary Cottam, *Radical Help: How We Can Remake the Relationships between Us and Revolutionise the Welfare State* (London: Hachette UK, 2018), 144.

an essential part of all medical care, the phenomenon is presently not part of scientific medicine. The reason is evident: it is a phenomenon that cannot be understood when health is reduced to mechanical functioning.[42]

Capra and Luisi make some crucial points in this quote. The first part could be looked at from a time-based perspective. They suggest that if the "medical researchers and practitioners" were to expand their scope to include the life conditions that lead up to the disease, that would be quite different from the relatively short-term perspective taken with this relatively simplistic 'interference' approach they described above.

The second point has to do with stepping back and widening the view, "from the level of organs and cells to the whole person."

The third point, regarding healing, further extends the scope of time into the future, and would seem to require something like patience: giving the body time and space to heal.

But their main point here is subtle. Healing is mysterious; it falls outside the bounds of totally controllable, predictable factors. It helps to be familiar with the principles of "certainty" versus "uncertainty" to understand their point. (See, for example, page 167 of Donella Meadows' book *Thinking In Systems: A Primer* for more.) This really is a worldview shift: from the supposed "certainty" we impose on living systems (including our own bodies) in an attempt to control outcomes, to a more

---

42   Fritjof Capra and Pier Luigi Luisi, *The Systems View of Life: A Unifying Vision* (Cambridge: Cambridge University Press, 2014), 323–24.

nuanced, artful approach that encompasses a much wider range of factors, and puts a certain level of trust in the unknown. Clearly we are no longer in the realm of command and control when it comes to the mystery of healing, and Capra and Luisi suggest we move deeper into that rather than ignore or try to override it, as our current medical model tends to do.

Health and Profit
Another serious challenge to health from a systems perspective is the profit motive.

In *The Healthcare Divide* from PBS's Frontline program, Dr. Chris Young, Chief of Staff at Erlinger Health System, a public hospital in Chattanooga, Tennessee says, "We talk a lot about *systems*, but the reality is we have a healthcare *marketplace*."[43]

In an extreme example of for-profit hospitals doing bad things (for-profit hospitals account for around 25% of hospitals in the U.S.), this same documentary referenced the case of Prospect Medical Holdings. This company took out over $1 billion in loans in 2018 and turned around and paid out $457 million of that money in dividends to investors.[44]

Brookings Institution, a nonprofit public policy organization, provides a high-level economic view of the medical industry in the United States:

---

43   Frontline PBS, Official, "The Healthcare Divide (Full Documentary) | FRONTLINE," YouTube, May 19, 2021, 16:40, https://www.youtube.com/watch?v=UVvEkeH4O8o.
44   Ibid., 44:40.

The health-care sector is in many ways the most consequen-
tial part of the United States economy . . . The health-care
sector now employs 11 percent of American workers . . . and
accounts for 24 percent of government spending . . . health-
care is one of the largest categories of consumer spending . . .
[. . .] Unfortunately, the problems with U.S. healthcare
are substantial. The United States spends more than other
countries without obtaining better health outcomes . . .
Sixty years ago, healthcare was 5 percent of the U.S. econ-
omy . . . at 17.7 percent in 2018, it was more than three
times that.[45]

Lack of a Common Social Ethic

A PBS Newshour episode interviewed Tsung-Mei Cheng, a
health policy analyst at Princeton University, who made it clear
why the United States healthcare system lags so far behind the
rest of the developed world, both in terms of outcomes and
exorbitant costs:

In this country we're very different from these other coun-
tries that have health insurance that covers everyone.
Health reformers in Europe [and] in Asia, they would
make explicit the social ethic that underlies that health
system . . . You say, what is it that we value, as a society?

---

45   Ryan Nunn, Jana Parsons, and Jay Shambaugh, "A Dozen Facts About
     the Economics of the Us Health-Care System," Brookings, March 10,
     2020, https://www.brookings.edu/research/a-dozen-facts-about-the-
     economics-of-the-u-s-health-care-system/.

*And then they build their healthcare system around that.
But in this country, because we have never been able to
achieve a social and political majority consensus, we live
with the status quo, which is that people who have insurance get care, and those who don't, don't.*[46]

In the United States—and certainly Marin County—we
have a situation where we allegedly think in terms of "healthcare" but the reality is more along the lines of medical industry
profit and growth. Note that Cheng is speaking about the "purpose" of a society and pointing to the capacity of other countries to land on some version of a shared purpose that enables
considerably better quality healthcare for their citizens than
that of the United States (and for dramatically lower cost).

What is "Health"?

"Health" is often thought of in the negative: as an *absence* of
disease and disorders, as opposed to the *presence* or prevalence
of well-being. It's easier to define health in the negative because
the presence of disorder tends to be more obvious and easier
to quantify than the presence of well-being. "Health" is also
one of the most general terms of the entire set of Sustainable
Development Goals. On top of that, measuring well-being is
at least as challenging as measuring health; perhaps more so.
We don't have a national well-being report on the level that
we have the *County Health Rankings & Roadmap* ratings.

---

46   PBS NewsHour, "Health Care: America vs. the World," YouTube, April
      22, 2021, 12:45, https://www.youtube.com/watch?v=BytzrjEfyfA.

For our purposes, we will fold "health" into well-being, but keep in mind that a person who has a serious medical condition—and therefore could be said to be "unwell"—could actually have a higher level of overall well-being than someone who fits your typical "healthy" profile. The latter may be suffering from less obvious, less tangible lifestyle factors that are harder to observe and quantify.

The SDG #3 Targets

We turn now to the larger picture of health, both globally and nationally, from the mainstream perspective. By "mainstream" I mean we will look at the data that is widely available and cited. This SDG has nine targets and two sub-targets. (I'm using the word "sub-targets" to indicate "3.A" and "3.B.").

Maternal and Infant Mortality
The first two targets under SDG #3 appear at first glance to be of less immediate concern in our "first world" setting:

3.1 By 2030, reduce the global maternal mortality ratio to less than 70 per 100,000 live births.

3.2 By 2030, end preventable deaths of newborns and children under 5 years of age, with all countries aiming to reduce neonatal mortality to at least as low as 12 per 1,000 live births and under-5 mortality to at least as low as 25 per 1,000 live births.

Experts say that "Maternal mortality is a key indicator of population health".[47] This makes the monitoring and reporting of maternal mortality a very important indicator in the health of our human system. It's a little bit like the canary in the coal mine.

But maternal mortality is a complex factor to measure, relying on administrative reporting by healthcare workers, all kinds of institutional databases and forms, not to mention coroner and autopsy reports, combined with records of pregnancy status, timing of death, etc. This is all extremely time consuming, and reliant on the allocation of public funds, with the support of NGO staff, to carry out these monitoring and reporting efforts.

According to the National Center for Health Statistics, in 2019 the number of maternity-related deaths reported country-wide was 754, or **20.1 per 100,000 live births**.[48] This puts the U.S. as a whole well below the "70 per 100,000 live births" SDG target.

However, the maternal mortality rate (the number of female deaths per 100,000 live births) for "Non-Hispanic black" women was 44 versus Hispanic women at 12.6, and "Non-Hispanic White" at 17.9. (These statistics are somewhat

---

47   California Pregnancy Mortality Surveillance System, "California Pregnancy-Related Deaths, 2008-2016" (California Pregnancy Mortality Surveillance System, 2021), 6, https://www.cdph.ca.gov/Programs/CFH/DMCAH/surveillance/CDPH%20Document%20Library/CA-PMSS/CA-PMSS-Surveillance-Report-2008-2016.pdf.

48   Donna L. Hoyert, "Maternal Mortality Rates in the United States, 2019" (National Center for Health Statistics, April 1, 2021), https://doi.org/10.15620/cdc:103855.

higher than 2018 data.) These numbers reflect the stark reality that African American women experience complications and even death during or related to childbirth at considerably higher rates than most other groups.

Unfortunately, Native North American women also have much higher maternal mortality rates than most other groups. The rates of disparity for both African American and Native North American women increase with age. See Figure 7 below.

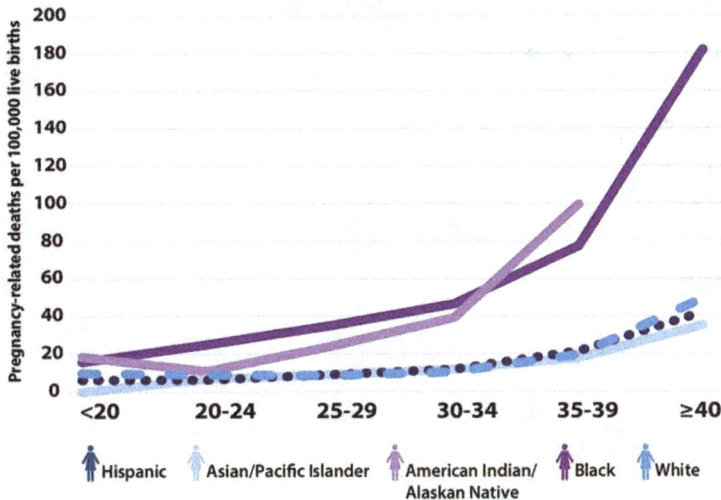

Figure 7 - CDC, "Racial/Ethnic Disparities in Pregnancy-Related Deaths" [49]

---

49   Center for Disease Control and Prevention, "Racial/Ethnic Disparities in Pregnancy-Related Deaths — United States, 2007–2016" (United States Government, 2017), 2, https://www.cdc.gov/reproductive-health/maternal-mortality/disparities-pregnancy-related-deaths/Infographic-disparities-pregnancy-related-deaths-h.pdf.

California

California's maternity death rate was 5.9 in 2016, compared to the national rate of 21.8 per 100,000 live births. That means California is doing quite well with regard to maternity death rates. One article cites a 55% decline in our state's maternal mortality rate from 2006 to 2013.[50] But that is not true for everyone.

According to *Maternity Care in California, 2019: A Bundle of Data,* Black women have long suffered a disproportionate share of maternal mortality (defined as 42 days or less postpartum).[51] See the chart below from this same study.

Maternal Mortality, by Race/Ethnicity
California, 2000 to 2013

MATERNAL DEATHS PER 100,000 LIVE BIRTHS

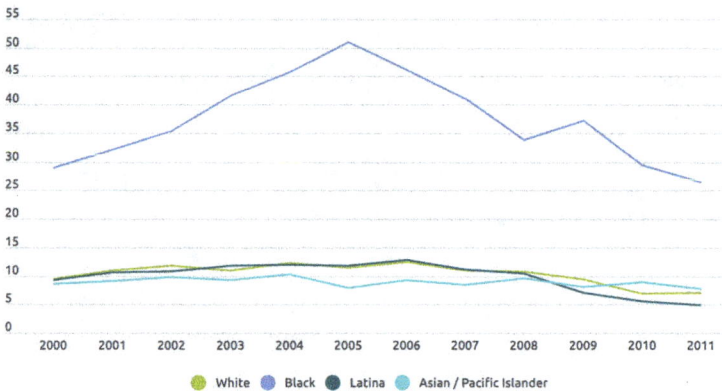

Figure 8 - California Health Care Foundation, 2018

---

50   Kyley Warren, "As Maternal Mortality Rises in U.S., California Bucks the Trend," Cronkite News, December 16, 2019, https://cronkitenews. azpbs.org/2019/12/16/california-maternal-mortality-rates/.

51   California Health Care Almanac, "Maternity Care in California, 2019: A Bundle of Data," 2019, https://www.chcf.org/wp-content/uploads/2019/11/MaternityCareCAAlmanac2019.pdf.

Marin County

In the 2019 *County Health Rankings* data, Marin County reported a total of three infant deaths (considered an infant within one year of age). Race is not reported. My assumption is that race is omitted at least in part to protect privacy, given the very small number of people. One can't help but wonder about the ethnicity and income level of those very few infant deaths.

Communicable & Non-Communicable Diseases

The next two health targets are related to diseases:

> *3.3 By 2030, end the epidemics of AIDS, tuberculosis, malaria and neglected tropical diseases and combat hepatitis, water-borne diseases and other communicable diseases.*

> *3.4 By 2030, reduce by one third premature mortality from non-communicable diseases through prevention and treatment and promote mental health and well-being.*

Note the language of "communicable" and "non-communicable" disease. Target 3.3 provides examples of "communicable" in its language. Examples of "non-communicable" are not listed out in 3.4, but cancer, heart disease, diabetes, and others are considered "non-communicable" diseases. We will continue looking at data related to this later group.

U.S. Healthcare (and the State of Our Health) is Not the Best

In case you have any illusions about us having pretty good overall health in the U.S., here are some examples to dispel that misinformation. (Note that there are slight variations in how these factors are measured. I chose one set of data, but you will find some differences from other sources.)

Longevity

According to the World Health Organization (WHO) and their 2019 data, **a child born today in the United States has a life expectancy of 78.5 years.**[52] That's almost six years less than the top life expectancy country, which is Japan, at 84.26 years. Of the 183 countries in the WHO's list, the U.S. is in 39th place. Turkey is right above us. With Croatia above them. And Estonia above them. Stereotypically some may view Colombia as a drug and gang-ridden, poverty-stricken country, but their lifespan is predicted to be almost a year longer than ours, at 79.31 years.

Overall Health

In overall health, the Bloomberg 2020 Global Health Index ranks **the U.S. as 35ᵗʰ** out of all countries included in the ranking.[53]

---

52   "Life Expectancy at Birth (Years)," accessed August 26, 2022, https://www.who.int/data/gho/data/indicators/indicator-details/GHO/life-expectancy-at-birth-(years).

53   "Bloomberg's Global Health Index for 2020," World Health, June 18, 2020, https://worldhealth.net/news/bloombergs-global-health-index-2020.

According to the "Cleanest Countries in the World 2022" report from the Yale / World Economic Forum "Environmental Performance Index," the United States does not make the top-ten cleanest countries in the world list.[54] Rather, out of a possible score of 100, the U.S. scores 69.3 for a cumulative total of rankings based on the cleanliness of our water and air, as well as our handling of waste and sanitation.

Healthcare Spending

There is one area in which the United States *is* first: spending on healthcare. According to the national Centers for Medicare and Medicaid Services, the total expenditure on healthcare in the U.S. was **$3.8 trillion in 2019**.[55] This is up 4.6 percent from 2018's total of $3.6 trillion. Virtually all healthcare spending at the country level is presented as per capita figures. The U.S. per capita spending is by far the highest, at $11,582 per person in 2019. In 2018 it was $10,948.

The closest country after the U.S. in terms of healthcare spending per capita is Switzerland, at $7,138 per person in 2018; that's about 65% of what we spend per person. (And yes, they rank well above the U.S., at #5 according to the Bloomberg 2020 Global Health Index cited above.)

---

54 "Cleanest Countries in the World 2022," World Population Review, accessed August 26, 2022, https://worldpopulationreview.com/country-rankings/cleanest-countries-in-the-world.

55 Micah Hartman et al., "National Health Care Spending in 2020: Growth Driven by Federal Spending in Response to the Covid-19 Pandemic: National Health Expenditures Study Examines Us Health Care Spending in 2020," *Health Affairs* 41, no. 1 (January 1, 2022): 13–25, https://doi.org/10.1377/hlthaff.2021.01763.

We have already reviewed lots of data. The way health data is done leaves out relationships and doesn't really account for well-being. Underneath it all, there is the pervasive specter of a profit-based "healthcare" system. We will continue with the numbers, and circle back to more of a systems view.

Epidemic of the Chronic

The year 2020 came along with the COVID-19 pandemic. The pandemic was made all the worse by the prevalence of chronic disease globally, which laid the ground for widespread suffering and death in the wake of COVID. COVID-19 is a "communicable" disease that, in essence, capitalized on the ripe ground for harvest set in place by *noncommunicable* disease. (Epidemiologists make use of this colorful, grim reaper term, "harvest," to indicate excessive deaths during a pandemic or other circumstances leading to a substantially increased number of deaths.)

The phrase "chronic disease" and noncommunicable disease sometimes seem to be used interchangeably, however, diseases such as AIDS are chronic, but also communicable. Chronic diseases include many disorders, including cancers, heart attacks and stroke, pulmonary diseases, Alzheimer's disease, and diabetes.

A 2022 article in *The Atlantic* profiles a long-standing trend of high rates of premature death among Americans, saying, "From 2019 to 2021, the number of working-age Americans who died [from COVID] increased by 233,000—and nine in 10 of those deaths wouldn't have happened if the U.S. had mortality rates on par with its peers".[56]

In short, the COVID-19 pandemic has been a sweeping instance of communicable disease meeting noncommunicable disease for a dramatic outcome.

Chronic Globe

According to the World Health Organization, 71% of all deaths globally (41 million people) are due to chronic disease.[57] Chronic disease is the leading cause of death (and disability) worldwide.

Chronic Nation

Chronic disease is also the leading cause of death here in the United States. But it's not only deaths that are the problem. It's also the psychological, social, financial burden of *living with* chronic disease. According to the U.S. Center for Disease Control (CDC), not only do **6 in 10 U.S. adults have a chronic disease**, but 4 in 10 have two or more.[58] If 60% of people in the U.S. have a chronic disease, this means *the majority of the population is unwell.* The CDC puts the annual healthcare cost of chronic disease at $3.8 trillion.

---

56 Ed Yong, "America Was in an Early-Death Crisis Long Before Covid," *The Atlantic*, July 21, 2022, sec. Health, https://www.theatlantic.com/health/archive/2022/07/us-life-span-mortality-rates/670591/.

57 "Non Communicable Diseases," World Health Organization, April 13, 2021, https://www.who.int/news-room/fact-sheets/detail/noncommunicable-diseases.

58 "Chronic Diseases in America," Centers for Disease Control and Prevention, May 6, 2022, https://www.cdc.gov/chronicdisease/resources/infographic/chronic-diseases.htm.

Note that the CDC's definition of chronic disease as appears on their website does not appear to include autoimmune disorders.[59] However, many autoimmune disorders can accurately be described as "chronic," in that they tend to be ongoing. They are also on the rise.[60]

Chronic California

According to the California Department of Public Health, "Chronic disease and injury are the leading causes of death, disability and diminished quality of life in California, and make up 80 percent of California's healthcare expenditures."[61]

Let's just pause for a moment. As we've already reviewed, chronic disease includes a number of very familiar health issues. The definition of the word "chronic" means something that lasts a long time or reoccurs periodically, repeatedly, over a long period of time. So, what this statistic is saying is that *the vast majority of spending in the medical sector goes to dealing with diseases that are technically preventable.*

59   "About Chronic Diseases," Centers for Disease Control and Prevention, July 21, 2022, https://www.cdc.gov/chronicdisease/about/index.htm.
60   Gregg E. Dinse et al., "Increasing Prevalence of Antinuclear Antibodies in the United States," *Arthritis & Rheumatology* 72, no. 6 (2020): 1026–35, https://doi.org/10.1002/art.41214.but findings are limited by the lack of systematic data and evolving approaches and definitions. This study was undertaken to investigate whether the prevalence of antinuclear antibodies (ANA
61   "Division of Chronic Disease and Injury Control," California Department of Public Health, February 8, 2018, https://www.cdph.ca.gov/Programs/CCDPHP/DCDIC/Pages/DivisionofChronicDiseaseandInjuryControl.aspx.

Are chronic diseases preventable? As a society we have a reasonable grasp on their causes. It's not absolute on a per-person basis; not remotely. But prosaic as it may sound, the CDC points to a very basic set of factors that have led to this extreme situation: tobacco use, poor nutrition, lack of physical activity, and excessive alcohol use.[62]

Marin County & Chronic Disease
We began this chapter with the factoid that Marin County consistently receives the highest health score out of all counties. But the highest out of what? If we're grading on a curve, we do great. But what if we're not?

---

62   "Chronic Diseases in America," Centers for Disease Control and Prevention, May 6, 2022, https://www.cdc.gov/chronicdisease/resources/infographic/chronic-diseases.htm.

Age-adjusted Death Rate by Chronic Disease, 2018, Marin
County and CA
Source: 2018 County Health Status Profiles, CDPH

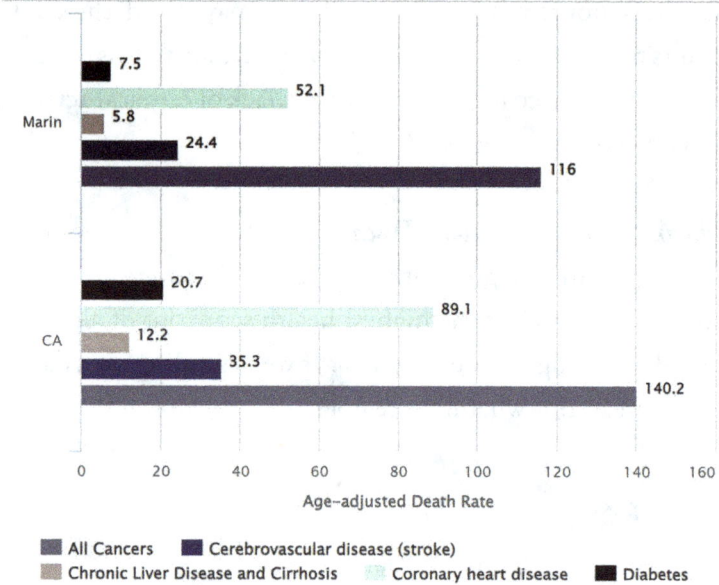

Figure 9 - Chronic Disease Rates in Marin County, FORWARD, 2018

What the bar chart above tells us is that, for example,
Marin County's "All Cancers" rate is 116 per 100,000 people,
while California's rate is 140.2 per 100,000 people. [63] Overall,
Marin County's rates of chronic disease are lower than the
state average, but we still have substantial occurrences of
chronic disease, and in proportions that closely mirror those
at the state level.

_____

63 "Chronic Disease Dashboard: Marin County," Livestories, accessed
    August 26, 2022, https://insight.livestories.com/s/v2/chronic-disease-
    dashboard-marin-county/545a68f2-34bd-4ba6-a0f5-c2b3433a67fb/.

In short, while our health outcomes are better than your average Californian, we have clearly not escaped the chronic disease trap here in Marin County.

Social Determinants of Health

You may want to check out "What do we know about social determinants of health in the U.S. and comparable countries?" on healthsystemtracker.org. But perhaps do that on a day when you're feeling resilient. If you are a United Statesian, it's going to make you feel awful about your country.

They explain, "This collection of charts explores international comparisons of social, environmental, and economic factors that influence health. . . " They go on to say, "Relative to similarly wealthy countries [12 of them], the U.S. has worse life expectancy, mortality, and disease burden rates, which may be due in part to the quality of care provided."[64]

Further charts illustrate stark realities. Both Black and White people have shorter life expectancies on average than in other economically comparable countries. We have the highest income disparities (using the "Gini coefficient"). Even in areas where we appear to be doing well—like lower cigarette smoking and alcohol drinking than comparable countries— we still have some of the worst outcomes, like higher rates of

---

64   Rabah Kamal, Cynthia Cox, and Erik Blumenkranz, "What Do We Know About Social Determinants of Health in the U.s. and Comparable Countries?," Peterson-KFF Health System Tracker, November 21, 2017, https://www.healthsystemtracker.org/chart-collection/know-social-determinants-health-u-s-comparable-countries/.

lung cancer and alcohol use disorders. (What's up with that?) We have a dramatically higher prevalence of obesity, the highest prevalence of cardiovascular diseases, and the highest rate of vehicle road injuries (517 per 100,000 people), with almost twice the rate of Canada, the next highest (287 per 100,000 people). Our "accidental poisonings," which includes drug overdoses, are far and away the highest of the 13 countries in the group.

The way they account for injuries and deaths due to firearms is complicated, but they summarize it by saying, "In the U.S. 225 years of life per 100,000 people are lost to disability and premature death as a result of assault by firearm – almost 19 times the comparable country average of 12 years of life per 100,000 people." In short, not surprisingly, deaths and injuries due to firearms in the U.S. are extreme, compared to the next closest country (again, Canada).

What do they mean by "225 years of life"? It's the result of adding up all of of the presumed years of "normal life" lost per 100 thousand people due to death or disability from firearms.

Disparities

Here are a few examples of what are often referred to as "disparities" between different racial, economic and social groups, as documented in the *County Health Rankings & Roadmaps* report of 2019.

In California, 12% of African American babies are born at what is called a "low birth weight," versus 6% of Hispanic and

5% of White babies.[65]

Teen birth rates among Hispanic females in 2019 was 29 teens per 1,000 females (aged 15-19), while the teen birth rate for African Americans was 12, and for Whites, 1.[66]

Their "Length of Life" measure is a bit confusing. It's essentially a "Premature death" score, and you want a low number. The number itself is described as "Years of Potential Life Lost Rate," further described as "Years of potential life lost before age 75 per 100,000 population (age-adjusted)."

In any case, these are the numbers in the 2019 report:

Black: 6,600
White: 3,200
Hispanic: 2,700

This shows that Black people have twice the number of "years of potential life lost" as Whites, and Hispanic people have the least years lost. (Data for 2018 and 2020, the year before and the year after, are similar.)

In Marin

The Measure of America has applied their well-being rubric to many communities in the United States, including Marin. They published a report for Marin County in 2012. (They released an update for California in 2021.) Their assessment

---

65 "Marin County, California," *County Health Rankings & Roadmaps*, 2019, https://www.countyhealthrankings.org/app/california/2019/rankings/marin/county/outcomes/overall/snapshot.
66 Ibid.

includes three overarching categories: a long and healthy life, access to knowledge, and a decent standard of living.[67] That report, *A Portrait of Marin,* is perhaps the most cited report I've run across in my five years of attending social equity meetings in the county. People tend to specifically reference the length of life difference and overall human development index differences (not just how long people tend to live, but all kinds of other factors related to well-being) between Ross at the top, and lower income neighborhoods at the bottom.

At the top of the chart (out of 48 census tracts) is Ross at 9.70. At the bottom is the Canal area of San Rafael, with an Index score of 3.18—below that of West Virginia, the lowest-ranked state on the American Human Development Index.[68]

---

67   Sarah Burd-Sharps and Kristen Lewis, "A Portrait of Marin: Marin County Human Development Report" (American Human Development Project of the Social Science Research Council, 2012), 18, http://www.measureofamerica.org/docs/APOM_Final-SinglePages_12.14.11.pdf.

68   Burd-Sharps and Lewis, 4.

		HD INDEX	LIFE EXPECTANCY AT BIRTH (years)
	California	5.54	80.1
	Marin County	7.75	83.7
1	Ross	9.70	88.0
2	Tiburon: Bel Aire	9.21	84.3
3	Tiburon: Downtown	9.08	83.4
4	Mill Valley: Old Mill, Cascade	9.00	82.8
5	Greenbrae	8.90	84.8
6	San Rafael: Glenwood, Peacock Gap	8.76	81.7
7	Sausalito	8.75	81.0
8	Tam Valley	8.73	80.9
9	Larkspur: Piper Park	8.71	84.0
10	Homestead Valley	8.70	80.6
41	Novato: Hamilton	6.52	75.2
42	Novato: Lynwood	6.47	80.1
43	Marin City	6.32	77.4
44	Novato: Olive–Deer Island	6.05	78.4
45	Novato: Downtown, Pioneer Park, San Marin	5.91	81.3
46	Nicasio, Point Reyes Station, Dillon Beach, Tomales	5.68	79.4
47	San Rafael: Santa Venetia	5.02	80.6
48	San Rafael: Canal Area	3.18	80.5

Figure 10 - Modified from Burd-Sharps and Lewis.

Keep in mind this data is over ten years old and to my knowledge the Index has not been updated for Marin County.

The report's Human Development Index scoring of various ethnic groups in Marin County is also confronting, showing that Asian and White ethnic groups score far higher in their Human Development Index and Life Expectancy in years than African Americans and Latinos. (We can infer that this report is an example of a report in which data for Native Americans is sparce and so they left out this group.)

	HD INDEX	LIFE EXPECTANCY AT BIRTH (years)
United States	**5.10**	78.6
California	**5.54**	80.1
Marin County	**7.75**	83.7
Asian Americans	**8.88**	90.9
Whites	**8.44**	83.5
African Americans	**5.72**	79.5
Latinos	**5.17**	88.2

Figure 11 – Variations by Race & Ethnicity in Marin County

As you can see, while the *County Health Rankings & Roadmaps* has consistently ranked Marin as the healthiest county in California, looking below the surface it becomes evident we reflect the same disparities and challenges as the rest of the state, and the country.

Where do we want to get to?

We need to be aiming our policies and programs toward meeting this Global Goal and the targets under it that are relevant to our community, as well as putting in place targets that capture our unique situation here in Marin.

In short, we want to "not" reflect the same disparities found in the state and the nation. We want to bring *everyone* up to the higher level of health experienced on average by people in

Marin, not leaving low-income and non-White racial groups subject to the same factors that suppress the well-being of people in other places. Further, we don't want factors here in Marin to lead to lower than average outcomes for low-income and non-White people.

World Happiness
In July 2011, the United Nations General Assembly adopted "UN Resolution 65/309 Happiness: Towards a Holistic Approach to Development".[69] This resolution put in motion the World Happiness Report (and a resolution the following year which declared that March 20th is henceforth the International Day of Happiness), which is run by the Sustainable Development Solutions Network. Gallup World Poll and several other partners and supporters make this report happen.

Shortly I will make a specific suggestion: putting mental health first is the way forward. Let's look a bit deeper at "happiness," and how it relates to mental health.

Happiness, Relationships, and Trust
I will not delve into the details of "affective" happiness versus "evaluative" happiness but suffice it to say that a cheap version of surface happiness is not at all what we mean here. Rather, the following quote from the 2021 *World Happiness Report* speaks to a view of happiness with depth:

69   United Nations, "Resolution Adopted by the General Assembly on 19 July 2011" (United Nations, August 19, 2011).

Trust and the ability to count on others are major supports to life evaluations, especially in the face of crises. To feel that your lost wallet would be returned if found by a police officer, by a neighbour, or a stranger, is estimated to be more important for happiness than income, unemployment, and major health risks.[70]

This is a very significant claim that gets to the core of the often overlooked (because hard to measure) factor of social ties at a community level. That is, resilient systems (in this case, communities) are those with the greatest number of connections. The fewer the connections, the more fragile (and unhappy) the system (or group of people).

Note that once again, this fundamentally important factor in human well-being centers on the strength of our *relationships* with one another.

Mental Health Toll of Poverty or "Happiness Inequality"
I learned this term, "happiness inequality," from Jon Clifton, CEO of Gallup, discussing the *2021 World Happiness Report.* While on the one hand we know that money doesn't fix all of your problems (a complex subject we will look at a bit more in the SDG #5 Gender equality chapter), on the other, there is a

---

70   John F. Helliwell et al., eds., *World Happiness Report 2021* (New York: Sustainable Development Solutions Network, 2021), https://happiness-report.s3.amazonaws.com/2021/WHR+21.pdf.

growing gap between wealthy and low-income groups in terms of self-reported quality of life measures. [71]

According to *Science,* "Within a given location, those with the lowest incomes are typically 1.5 to 3 times more likely than the rich to experience depression or anxiety."[72] In short, how can we avoid the trap of "Happiness Inequality" in Marin County?

How do we get there?

We have established some basis for the claim that the purpose of the system we call "healthcare" in the United States is actually "sick care" for the purposes of profit and growth. If we would prefer to have a robust system of care for people suffering various ailments, and a robust system of tending wellness overall, then what has to change?

Do we need better policies? Better programs? More money?

Just as with the other Global Goals, it seems as though despite all of our efforts and money and wringing of hands, the situation is getting worse. Why? Because the purpose of the overall system—its primary function—is to produce profit. If its primary function was to promote and support well-being, holy-gosh we would have a very different system from the one we have today.

---

71   SDSN, "Launch of the 2021 World Happiness Report," YouTube, March 23, 2021, 07:07, https://www.youtube.com/watch?v=Xi7ok0xzzqE.

72   Matthew Ridley et al., "Poverty, Depression, and Anxiety: Causal Evidence and Mechanisms," *Science* 370, no. 6522 (December 11, 2020): eaay0214, https://doi.org/10.1126/science.aay0214.

If the question of purpose attends to the "what," then what is the "how"? That is, how do we attend to the "how" we get to where we want to be?

If we take the insights of Hillary Cottam and her team's work in the UK, we can see that policy, programs and money all play a part, but if the so-called "solutions" ignore the central importance of relationships, nothing will work.

The challenging reality is that as a county, Marin only has so much control over its collective level of health. Sure, we come out on top right now in terms of averages, but as we have covered, that is due to the "wealth equals health" phenomenon (which is both an inaccurate and accurate claim, depending on what you do or don't measure).

Our national healthcare system is lagging behind the rest of the developed world in terms of quality health outcomes, while at the same time is much higher than the rest of the world in terms of cost. This is something you can roll with if you are wealthy. But if you are not, the stresses become exponential.

So given this collective reality, where should we focus? The answer: mental health.

Mental Health

Why mental health? Let's presume for a moment that "health" is a subsystem of "well-being." Well-being is much larger than physical health. A case could be made that well-being and mental health are the same. But for our purposes let's say that well-being encompasses but is not limited to mental health.

We therefore have these three categories, decreasing in size in terms of scope:

- **Well-being**
- Mental health
- Physical health

What most people mean by "health" is physical health. How do we know? If I say to you, "How has your health been lately?" you're going to reflexively think about your blood pressure, weight, whether or not you have had a cold or flu (or COVID), etc. Mental health is often an afterthought; adjacent to, but not top-of-mind when the topic of "health" arises.

The phrase "mental health" encompasses a lot. It's not only conditions such as depression and schizophrenia that are covered by this term, but also addiction, social connection, and spiritual health.

With a brief thought experiment you can see that, generally speaking, if you have good mental health but poor physical health, you have a much better chance of getting through with a higher level of well-being than if the reverse is true. That is, if you have poor mental health, your level of overall well-being is much more fragile.

Let's not be overly simplistic here. Physical maladies can and do take a tremendous psychological toll, creating a rein-forcing feedback loop of suffering. Nevertheless, your chances of recovery, or of dealing well with death and dying are much improved when your psychological well-being—mental health—is amply resourced.

I am suggesting that mental health is in fact:

1. Somewhat more important and comprehensive than physical health
2. A close, though not exact synonym for "well-being."

There are two more reasons I think that mental health should be put first when it comes to realizing SDG #3 by 2030:

1. It is more easily measured and consistently tracked than well-being
2. It is currently the subject of stigma.

In the longer-term, doing the hard work of measuring and improving well-being is where we need to head. In the near-term, a focus on mental health is a great leap forward.

Plus, there is data that supports the link between psychological distress and developing disorders such as cancer. The American Association for Cancer Research looked at cancer mortality in the U.S. between 1997 and 2014. They found that "cancer mortality risk was 33 percent higher in adults with serious psychological distress compared to adults without psychological distress"[73]. That is a big difference.

What does it look like to put mental health *first* in our community?

---

73 "The State of Cancer Health Disparities in 2022," American Association for Cancer Research, accessed November 27, 2022, https://cancerprogressreport.aacr.org/disparities/cdpr22-contents/cdpr22-the-state-of-cancer-health-disparities-in-2022/.

The Marin Context

Elberta Eriksson was a licensed Marriage and Family Therapist (among other qualifications) and had been for her whole career. She was a long-term resident of Mill Valley serving her Southern Marin community for the past many decades of her life, specifically low-income families in Marin City. She passed away in 2022 at the age of 92.

Elberta promoted what she called a "wrap-around approach to social services," using the wrap-around term to refer not just to troubled youth (as the term officially refers to programs for youth in the foster care system), but to all individuals and families. In an effort to provide more quality services to a greater number of individuals, Elberta supervised graduate students in psychology working to earn their license since approximately 2010. The program is called the Southern Marin Community Connection.

Elberta had seen so many "new and exciting" programs come to town over the years that by the time I started supporting her group in 2018 she was down-right suspicious. She had a right to be. Philanthropy tends to favor the newest great idea, brought by the latest newcomers. Due to local politics, baggage, and our basic human propensity to get excited about the novel, philanthropy is better set up to provide short rather than long-term support. This means that programs like Elberta's fall off of the radar and tend to flounder, especially when the leader starts to be seen as saying the same ole' thing.

Elberta would often harken unto her version of the good ole' days and an organization she was an integral part of,

Operation Give A Damn (OGAD). You can refer to the blog on the Systems Thinking Marin website for more details about OGAD. Suffice it to say here that OGAD was a beautiful example of a community coming together to foster and build more and stronger social connections among people who needed extra support and people who could provide that for them, made possible by relatively small-scale funding. In a word, OGAD excelled at creating relationships.

The Family Functioning Scale

Trained in Family Systems with a good bit of systems thinking in the mix, Elberta's professional practice was what I call "systems'ey." In particular, she has developed the Family Functioning Scale, a qualitative scale (with a quantitative assessment component) that allows practitioners to holistically assess the well-being of their clients across eleven areas of life. From food and housing security to transportation, income and education and more, the Family Functioning Scale is a tool that is handed to the client for self-report and reflection and supplies a basis for shared discussion between client and provider.

As Justine Reese, a mental health provider who trained under Elberta, stated in one of Elberta's organizing meetings (the Southern Marin Multi-Disciplinary Team monthly meeting or MDT), "The mental health issues experienced by many of my clients are due to stressors in some other area of life, like income or housing." As a mental health service provider for low-income individuals in particular, it is simply impractical to limit your scope of support to the realm of mental health, strictly speaking. Justine and others in her position often find themselves devoting time beyond scheduled sessions to finding additional support services for clients; time for which they may not be paid, but which they see as crucial to the overall well-being and health of the person they are striving to support. It may be practical or impractical to limit the scope of your focus, but in either case, it's a factor of care and relationship-building that many practitioners go the extra mile to serve their clients. (Perhaps it goes without saying that practitioners who go the extra mile should be compensated and otherwise supported in providing this "wrap-around"-type support.)

Challenges With the Current Mental Health System

A quick aside: the current mental health system in Marin (and the United States, and possibly the Western world) is—like the "sick system"—lousy. I'm making a few claims here that come from conversations with people who are care providers in this system. (See Appendix A.) Funding for prevention is little or nonexistent. Low-income individuals suffer additional trauma from the humiliation of being treated like cogs in a machine when they are already at their lowest. And whether you are low, middle or high-income, society has made a fairly strict specialization out of mental health professionals while in subtle and overt ways discriminating against people suffering from mental health challenges. I suggest that if mental health, happiness and well-being overall were to be more closely equated, some of these unfortunate traps could be overcome.

Specific Ideas

As with the other chapters, the Introduction of this book provides an outlined set of general steps for organizing a holistic, community-based effort to harness existing local efforts and bring about much greater mutual coordination to reach a certain Global Goal. Given what we have covered so far, here are some specifics for #3 Good Health and Well-Being:

- County-wide adoption of Elberta Erkisson's Family Functioning Scale for individual, family, and even whole community reference and publicly-reported metrics
- Development of a service referral database so that practitioners such as Justine have a much easier time referring their clients to additional support services.
    - This has been tried again and again, across the country. Current national versions exist but something doesn't quite coagulate fully with all of them. The work of Open Referral and Greg Bloom is a great place to start; they have invested a lot of time in working out how this could possibly work.
- And finally, within the realm of SDG #3, put mental health first. As reviewed earlier in this chapter, mental health is a slightly more specific way of saying "well-being" (and even "happiness") and edges out other topics in terms of its outsized impact across all areas of well-being.

In summary, a coalition of organizations and individuals passionate about health and well-being in Marin County—those who are low-income and those who live as a part of low-income communities, whether they themselves are low-income or not—must come together. The work is to develop shared resources, timelines, and strategies. I make a case for placing mental health as the number one focus. But perhaps your in-depth interviews with community members and providers will reveal a different top-level focus? **Don't neglect to include a timeline for your local targets**; without a timeline for meeting targets, we can expect a lot of busy work and no real change.

CHAPTER 4

SDG #4 Quality Education

Where are we?

It's hard to look at Marin County's education system and *not* make your way rather quickly to topics related to some rather serious social equity issues. From a distance this would not seem to be the case. The tens of thousands of people who contributed to the creation of the SDGs were probably not too concerned with places such as Marin. This is underscored by statistics such as the following.

Marin's Educational Outcomes

The website Niche.com provides a list of "Counties with the Best Public Schools in California" for 2022, based on "state test scores, graduation rates, SAT/ACT scores, teacher quality, and student and parent reviews."[74] It's not a big shocker that Marin is #1. That means, statistically speaking, of all counties in California, your child has the best chance of getting a top-quality public education in Marin.

California's Educational Outcomes

While Marin ranks at the top of the heap within California, California itself ranks low among the 50 states for public school quality. This changes somewhat depending on what list you look to.

---

74   "2022 California Counties with the Best Public Schools," Niche, accessed August 26, 2022, https://www.niche.com/places-to-live/search/counties-with-the-best-public-schools/s/california/.

U.S. News and World Report ranks California #20 for state education systems, though, as of this writing, they don't make it obvious what they are relying on for that ranking.[75] Further, in their list of how well states prepare students for college, California ranks #40.[76]

Another rating system, provided by schoolaroo.com, ranks California #44 out of all 50 states .[77] As a systems thinker, I appreciate the fact that this ranking includes student safety, as this indicates a more holistic perspective.

(If you happen to run across alecreportcard.org for state educational rankings, keep in mind that this organization— and thus their ranking system—is undergirded by libertarian values and an exclusively Republican membership. Clearly, if you identify as Libertarian or Republican, you may find this site helpful.)

United States Educational Outcomes

U.S. News and World Report ranked the United States #1 in their "Best Countries for Education" list.[78] However, the Programme for International Student Assessment (PISA), a global study by the Organization for Economic Co-operation

---

75   "Best States for Education," US News, accessed August 26, 2022, https://www.usnews.com/news/best-states/rankings/education.

76   Estrella Rosas, "States with Best & Worst Public School Systems," Scholaroo, January 12, 2022, https://scholaroo.com/state-education-rankings/.

77   Ibid.

78   "Best Countries for Education," US News, accessed August 26, 2022, https://www.usnews.com/news/best-countries/best-countries-for-education.

and Development (OECD), paints a different picture. In the three PISA categories, the United States ranks well below many other OECD and non-OECD nations in these test performance areas:

Reading: #13
Science: #19
Math: #38[79]

Of course, test scores in reading, science and math only tell a portion of the story when it comes to one's ability to thrive in the world as an adult, which is why rankings of education systems do not usually rely on test scores alone. (We won't even get into the issue of country-based reporting shenanigans, that is, countries that want to look good in international rating systems, so they cherry-pick their best schools to participate in the survey.)

Socio-Economic Disparity in Education

Understanding where we are in Marin with regard to #4 Quality Education means looking at the economics of educational access. As with the first three SDGs, access to quality education—and thus educational outcomes—largely follow economic lines.

It is important to not allow jargon to obscure this basic fact: families with greater access to money have significantly

---

79 "Programme for International Student Assessment," in *Wikipedia*, August 5, 2022, https://en.wikipedia.org/w/index.php?title=Programme_for_International_Student_Assessment&oldid=1102460958.

greater access to quality education. Families with lesser access to money have an uphill battle. As we will see, Marin County is by no means exempt from this basic, collective reality.

A study by Stanford University and the group Policy Analysis for California Education, documents the following:

> ... *when California's scores are disaggregated by socioeconomic status (SES), affluent districts do score as well as similarly affluent districts in the rest of the country, while in nonaffluent districts, students score nearly a full grade level behind their peers nationwide...* [80]

These outcomes are not relegated to *academic* achievement. In a unique study by the OECD, "Beyond Academic Learning: First results from the survey of social and emotional skills," the author's state:

> *Students from advantaged backgrounds reported higher social and emotional skills than their disadvantaged peers in every skill that was measured and in all cities participating in the survey.*[81]

80   Harry Brighouse et al., "Outcomes and Demographics of California's Schools" (Stanford University, September 2018), 6, https://gettingdowntofacts.com/sites/default/files/2018-09/GDTFII_Brief_OutcomesandDemographics.pdf.
81   Organisation for Economic Co-operation and Development, *Beyond Academic Learning: First Results from the Survey of Social and Emotional Skills* (Paris: Organisation for Economic Co-operation and Development, 2021), 6, https://doi.org/10.1787/92a11084-en.

The social and emotional skills measured were based on five broad categories, Openness, Conscientiousness, Extraversion, Agreeableness and Neuroticism.[82] We will look at this report a bit more.

Native Americans & Education in California

An ABC News article cites Ed Data (ed-data.org) regarding educational outcomes for Native American and Alaskan Native youth in California Schools. It is a grim picture: Native Americans are least likely to graduate (75% graduation rate versus 85% for all students), least likely to meet UC/CSU requirements upon graduation (31% versus about half of all students), and have among the lowest test scores for English and Math.[83] The Postsecondary National Policy Institute cites that about 24% of Native Americans aged 18 – 24-years-old are enrolled in college, compared to 41% for the overall U.S. population.[84]

English Language Learners in Schools

According to the Public Policy Institute of California, nearly 25% of students in our state's schools are English Learners, but

---

82   Ibid., 20.

83   Grace Manthey and Christiane Cordero, "Indigenous Students Can Face Large Education Gaps. Here's How One School Is Trying to Close Them," ABC7 Los Angeles, November 24, 2021, https://abc7.com/native-american-education-indigenous-students-achievement-gaps-school/11263264/.

84   "Native American Students," Postsecondary National Policy Institute, November 17, 2021, https://pnpi.org/native-american-students/.

English Learners struggle to keep up academically with their peers for whom English is their native language.[85]

However, a growing body of research demonstrates that bilingual ability improves brain function: "The cognitive control required to manage multiple languages appears to have broad effects on neurological function, fine-tuning both cognitive control mechanisms and sensory processes."[86] According to a 2017 report from the bipartisan research and advocacy group New American Economy, the demand for bilingual jobs (both low and high-paying) has been on the upswing in recent years.[87] And people with disabilities are shown to not only be just fine with bilingualism, but in some cases being multilingual helps support their well-being.[88]

This is a classic case of an opportunity to turn a perceived disadvantage—a language other than English as a first language—into an advantage. And, this is an advantage that would benefit the entire community. With such a high percentage of English Learners in the public school system, along

85 "California's English Learner Students," Public Policy Institute of California, September 2012, https://www.ppic.org/publication/californias-english-learner-students/.

86 Viorica Marian and Anthony Shook, "The Cognitive Benefits of Being Bilingual," *Cerebrum: The Dana Forum on Brain Science* 2012 (October 31, 2012): 13.

87 "Demand for Bilingual Workers More Than Doubled in 5 Years, New Report Shows," New American Economy, March 1, 2017, https://www.newamericaneconomy.org/press-release/demand-for-bilingual-workers-more-than-doubled-in-5-years-new-report-shows/.

88 Izzy Bloom, "When You Don't Learn Your Parent's Language, What Is Lost?," KQED, May 20, 2002, https://www.kqed.org/news/11914760/when-you-dont-learn-your-parents-language-what-is-lost.

with the benefits of bilingual education, educating every child in California in both English and Spanish would seem a natural evolution with benefits for all involved.

A necessary distinction to note is that there are differences between being bilingual, biliterate, and bicultural. Having an in-depth relationship to another culture is a level above and beyond language.

Segregated Schools in Marin County?

Getting back to Marin, you will note a pattern repeating itself here. Marin has a high *average* within the state context. But the unfortunate reality is that some schools—and school children—are left in the dust.

Sausalito Marin City School District

One of our most extreme local examples of inequality within Marin came into the news in October 2018. Following a two-year investigation, the California State Attorney General ruled that the Sausalito Marin City School District illegally segregated their two community schools: Willow Creek Academy, a charter school in Sausalito, and Bayside Martin Luther King Jr., an elementary school a mile-and-a-half up the road in Marin City. It was the first desegregation order in California in over 50 years.

In what has come to be known as the "unification" process, since 2019 the two schools have been in a process of merging.[89]

---

89   Dana Goldstein and Anemona Hartocollis, "'Separate Programs for Separate Communities': California School District Agrees to Desegregate," *The New York Times*, August 9, 2019, sec. U.S., https://www.nytimes.com/2019/08/09/us/sausalito-school-segregation.html.

The new school (with two campuses) is called Dr. Martin Luther King, Jr. Academy.

I participated mid-stream, around October and November of 2021, in the unification efforts. At the practical level that looked like attending at least two public meetings, as well as participating in several "Process Committee" group meetings. There were five people in our group, and I was the newest to the issue, and therefore the least informed. It also meant that I brought the least baggage.

The major issue that was discussed in our small group was what two committee members called "family flight." They were concerned that families were and would continue to leave the district, taking their kids with them, due to how the district was handling funding of the two schools and perhaps other issues.

The other two participants were more concerned about current and historical racism in the district and seemed to feel that the "family flight" topic was blown out of proportion.

From the outset it became clear to me that these participants had history amongst themselves; contentious history that our little discussion committee was not equipped to handle sufficiently. As the facilitator, I ensured our short report back to the Superintendent was completed, sectioning out the two sides of the issue to highlight the on-going disagreement. We also included the following statement (which to my knowledge is not publicly available and therefore I do not have a citation for it):

#2: Addressing Division Head-On
Based on our observations and experience, this particular community faces exceptional uphill work to achieve the

"unity" ideal. Marin County has a documented history of racial and economic stratification, and that reality is the backdrop against which this process is playing out. We have division in the community--including in our own group--about what the facts are surrounding this process and history, and which next steps are most important.

If you are located in the district or have been watching local media, as you can see, controversy continues, in particular focused on Itoco Garcia. Garcia has been the Superintendent of the Board for this district through both COVID and the unification / desegregation process.

Marin County's Many Districts

Just to back up for a moment, Marin County has (believe it or not) eighteen school districts. Having a district (as opposed to just having a school) for your town means you keep your local property tax dollars in your own town's schools. Obviously, this is great for wealthy communities, and vice versa, not so great for neighboring less-wealthy communities.

If you don't have school-age children (or even if you do), you may not know that the hierarchy looks something like this:[90]

1. School Board (of a given district)
2. Superintendent of the District
3. Principal of a School Within a District

---

90   "Public School District (United States)," Ballotpedia, accessed August 28, 2022, https://ballotpedia.org/Public_school_district_ (United_States).

Local funding stays within this district structure. In other words, a very small, wealthy district in one area of Marin County does not share dollars in any fashion that I am aware of with middle or low-income districts in other parts of the county.

Where Schools Get Their Funding
When it comes to education, funding matters. From a systems thinking perspective, Donella Meadows' "Success to the Successful" principle or "trap" (covered in the Introduction) comes down hard in this area. It's not a surprise to see that schools that are well funded have much higher educational outcomes than schools that are poorly funded. Therefore, students whose families can afford to buy a home in a wealthier area are more likely to be able to send their kids to well-funded public schools (not to mention private schools), because the local property tax revenue is only going to their district's schools.

We're going to look at some examples of Marin school district funding. However, I want to acknowledge that funding for schools is a national, not just a local matter. How we do and don't prioritize school funding in our larger society impacts our local picture. I hit the roof every time I get an email asking me to donate to my niece or nephew's school; I blow off steam and then make a small donation. Then I curse our society that puts children and their families in the position of having to raise money to function.

Marin School Funding – Two Contrasting Examples

Marin Promise Partnership has a helpful graphic on their website that illustrates sources of school funding.[91] Note that locating documentation of, and then understanding school funding is a dramatic barrier to understanding how your local schools are actually funded; we have a lot of room to improve in this regard. The graphics provided by Marin Promise Partnership are a window in.

Beginning with their "ADA (Average Daily Attendance) Funding by District" infographic for their "Elementary School District Over 1k" segment of the local schools, we will look at two contrasting examples. These are numbers for the 2018 – 19 academic year. Both examples are drawn from both the "ADA Funding by District" and "Total Funding" tabs of the source website.

The Mill Valley district is shown to have a student population in which 7% of children in attendance are listed as "in Need," which they define in the fine print as "those classified as English learners, those meeting income or categorical eligibility criteria for participation in the National School Lunch Program, foster youth, or any combination of these factors."

---

91   "Funding Equity Initiative," Marin Promise Partnership, 2018, https://www.marinpromisepartnership.org/funding-equity-initiative/.

Mill Valley District

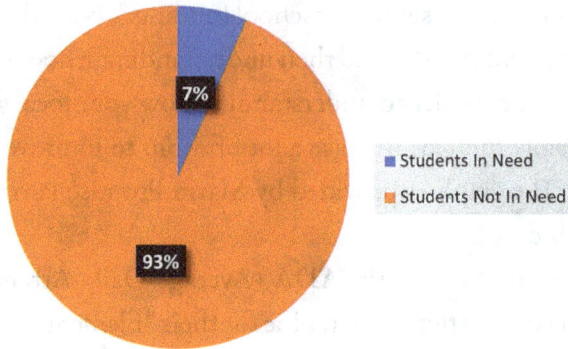

Figure 12 – Mill Valley District, 2018-19 Academic Year

The second, contrasting example we will look at is their "San Rafael City Elementary" school district, in San Rafael. In this district, 68% of students are defined as Students in Need.

San Rafael City Elementary

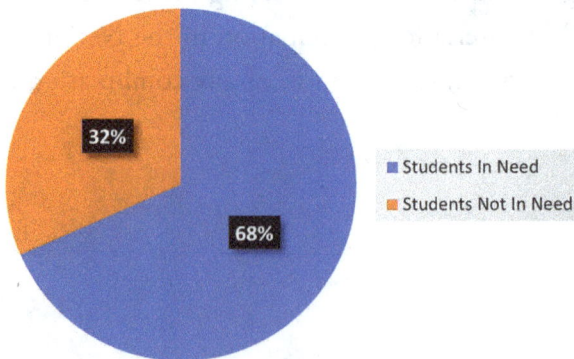

Figure 13 - San Rafael City Elementary, 2018-19 Academic Year

So, clearly the Mill Valley district has a proportionally far smaller group of "Students In Need" than the San Rafael district in this example. Further, looking at the total funding versus the total number of students illustrates that the Mill Valley district has nearly $3,000 in funding more *per year per student*.

- Mill Valley District, 2018 – 19 Academic Year
  - 2,979 students
  - $47.2 million
  - $15,844 per student
- San Rafael City Elementary District, 2018 – 19 Academic Year
  - 4,587 students
  - $59.6 million
  - $12,993 per student

Let's add in a couple of numbers.

The infographic reports the "Median Household Income" for the Mill Valley School District as $159,000.

In the San Rafael district, the Median Household Income is reported as $87,000.

If we stopped right there, we would see a dramatic negative correlation between percentage of Students in Need and Median Household Income: Mill Valley families make more money, and so of course have far fewer Students in Need in their district schools, as noted above. It is noteworthy that while Mill Valley families have a median household income of nearly *twice* that of their neighbors seven miles north, the San

Rafael City Schools district has almost *ten times* the number
of Students in Need.

The nearly $3,000 less per student in the San Rafael dis-
trict is particularly concerning in that many of the Students in
Need are, well, *in need*: in need of more resources, not fewer.
Revisiting the definition of this term, that means people learning English, receiving funding for lunch, people in the foster
system, "or any combination of these factors."

Visiting the "Total Funding" tab on the Marin Promise
website reveals pie graphs depicting the sources of that revenue.

Mill Valley District - Academic Year 2018 - 19

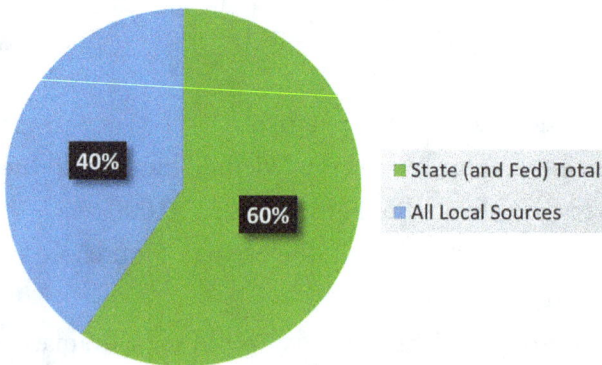

Figure 14 - Mill Valley District Funding

The Mill Valley District received 24% or $11.4 million
in Parcel Tax Funding in the 2018 – 19 school year. The less

affluent area of San Rafael's K-12 district received a much smaller percentage of their total budget from local property taxes; 5% for a total of $3.1 million.

San Rafael City Elementary - Academic Year 2018 - 19

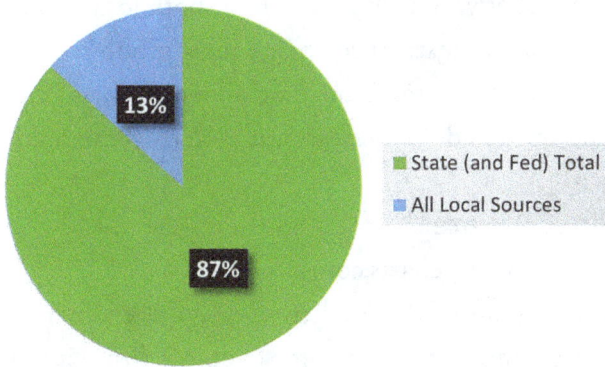

Figure 15 - San Rafael District Funding

What these two contrasting pictures show us is pretty obvious. First, local property taxes are not the *main* sources of funding for these two districts. Nevertheless, the much higher property value in the more affluent district is a much larger part of the pie in their total funding. The district with lower property values and less affluent families relies dramatically on state funding.

If you flip through the other graphs available on the Marin Promise Partnership website, you will see this general trend played out: affluent areas receiving a large chunk of their funding from local revenues; less affluent schools—often just a few miles up the road—relying for an even greater portion of their budget on state sources.

Our eighteen school districts with separate budgets simply means that *wealthier neighborhoods are not sharing with lower income neighborhoods.* This reinforces segregation (given the correlation between income and race) both locally and in our larger social context. At least one local group is organizing around attempts to combine some of our school districts. You can find them and their research at bettertogethermarin.org.

Public vs Private

According to towncharts.com (which cites the 2020 American Community Survey data as their source) one-quarter of Marin County's youth attend private schools.[92] (The only nearby county with a higher percentage of private school attendees is San Francisco, with 32%, or nearly 1/3 of their kids in private schools.) Marin's number is ten percentage points higher than California's, where overall 14% of our youth attend private institutions.

The National Assessment of Educational Progress (NAEP) assesses and reports on educational outcomes for both public and private schools. A 2021 U.S. News and World Report article states, "The most recent NAEP data shows what other

---

92   "Marin County California Education Data for Research San Francisco County and Sonoma County," Town Charts, accessed August 26, 2022, https://www.towncharts.com/California/Education/Marin-County-CA-Education-data.html.

research has found: Private school students score better in almost all subjects."[93]

However, the article goes on to cite research that points to a combination of the education level of parents and their income level being a better determiner of test scores than public versus private schools. They also point to evidence that low-income students at private schools, though their tests scores are somewhat below their higher income peers, the low-income student's educational outcomes are often above those of their public school peers:

> ... both types of students ... were less likely than traditional public school students to ever fail a course, or to ever be suspended in high school, and they were more likely to enroll in college within one year of high school graduation.

Keep in mind of course that studies such as this report averages, whereas outcomes will vary depending on the specific institution.

Where do we want to get to?

First, while I am proposing a few ideas here, the most important ideas would have to come from local youth in the school system, and adults who have grown up in it: in-depth conversations, over time, with a diversity of Marin County individuals

---

93 "Private School vs. Public School," US News & World Report, accessed August 28, 2022, //www.usnews.com/education/k12/articles/private-school-vs-public-school.

to find out what their experiences are, and what their aspirations are for their own lives.

Turning back to the OECD report, "Beyond Academic Learning: First results from the survey of social and emotional skills," the researchers document this important observation:

A striking, but not unexpected, result from the survey is that all 15-year-old students, irrespective of their gender and social background, reported lower social and emotional skills on average than their 10-year-old counterparts. Parent and educator ratings confirmed the dip in social and emotional skills as students grow older. Also, students' creativity and curiosity were found to be lower among 15-year-olds than 10-year-olds.[94]

They go on to speculate why this may be the case:

While developmental factors may play a role here, this might also partly derive from the fact that education systems often expect students to be compliant, which in turn may have the potential consequence of driving out curiosity and creativity as students grow older and stay longer in the education system.[95]

---

94   Organisation for Economic Co-operation and Development, *Beyond Academic Learning: First Results from the Survey of Social and Emotional Skills* (Organisation for Economic Co-operation and Development, 2021), 3, https://doi.org/10.1787/92a11084-en.

95   Ibid.

As a proponent of systems thinking, I can't tell you how many people I've spoken with who claim a parallel trend: they believe children to be "naturally systems thinkers," but feel that conventional education (and later, the standard work environment) reduces their ability to see the big picture. I believe this goes right along with the findings and speculations of the report cited above.

In light of this, I propose that we want to "get to" a different scenario; one in which students at 15 have improved upon the emotional skills, curiosity, and creativity of their 10-year-old selves.

Clearly, we also want income level and race to *not* predict educational *or* quality of life outcomes. This would mean that we see disparities in educational metrics close entirely. It would require that citizens of the more affluent towns learn to share with their lower income neighbors, fully and openly reflecting the fact that we are all in this together. Meeting SDG #4 Quality Education for All by 2030 in Marin County is probably one of the more accessible SDGs for us here locally. Nevertheless, closing the gaps 100% is a big hill to climb. It would require that every parent in Marin County extend their circle of compassion to include the children of their neighbors, most particularly including the Marin County neighbors they may not know personally, and who are not part of their socio-economic group.

Systems Thinking in Education

The argument for including systems thinking throughout education is made by The Worldwatch Institute in *Earth Ed:*

Rethinking Education on a Changing Planet.

> *How can education—whether in school, on a farm, in a lab, or at the kitchen table—enable the next generation to live sustainably and navigate the radical changes that they are inheriting in this human-dominated epoch? . . . Common sense tells us that to understand human impact on Earth's systems, we need to understand systems.[96]*

This takes us back to the point earlier in this chapter that we have qualities early in our development that are unfortunately either simply ignored or even actively diminished by our educational, social context.

How do we get there?

We've spent a lot of time in this chapter examining the current state of affairs, with the presumption that we want to get everyone to the same, high level depicted by the highest educational outcomes of the highest earning families at the best-performing schools.

However, there is an unexamined assumption here that needs to be examined: are schools working? Do we really want to bring "under achieving" students up to "achieving" in a system that is, overall, perhaps not serving our society particularly well?

---

96   Erik Assadourian, Lisa Mastny, and Worldwatch Institute, eds., *EarthEd: Rethinking Education on a Changing Planet*, State of the World (Washington, DC: Island Press, 2017), 145.

The Drop-Off

Mirroring the OECD's "Beyond Academic Learning" report cited above, research points to a dramatic drop-off in student engagement as they advance through their school systems.

A Gallup Poll from 2015 cites that about a third of 11th graders feel "engaged by school," whereas 75% of fifth-grade students report feeling engaged.[97] That is another example of a drop-off.

A 2019 New York Times article cites the work of two investigators who traveled across the country shadowing students at thirty different high schools, and published their findings in a book, *In Search of Deeper Learning: The Quest to Remake the American High School.*

> *... we noticed that powerful learning was happening most often at the periphery — in electives, clubs and extracurriculars. Intrigued, we turned our attention to these spaces. We followed a theater production. We shadowed a debate team. We observed elective courses in green engineering, gender studies, philosophical literature and more.*

> *As different as these spaces were, we found they shared some essential qualities. Instead of feeling like training grounds or holding pens, they felt like design studios or research*

97   Ross Brenneman, "Gallup Student Poll Finds Engagement in School Dropping by Grade Level," *Education Week*, March 23, 2016, sec. Families & the Community, https://www.edweek.org/leadership/gallup-student-poll-finds-engagement-in-school-dropping-by-grade-level/2016/03.

*laboratories: lively, productive places where teachers and
students engaged together in consequential work.*[98]

It's a bit of a strange experience to read this type of information, meaning, "No duah!" It's a little bit like, "Scientists
demonstrate a link between smoking cigarettes and lung
disease." But it does, in fact, appear as though we have been
so brainwashed into thinking of school as boring, nearly as a
necessary evil, that we have allowed generations upon generations of youth to suffer through half-baked and downright bad
school systems for at least a hundred years. (And we shouldn't
forget the teachers and administrators who are likewise
trapped in this industrial era system.)

Envision Schools

In the book *Transforming Schools: Using Project-Based
Learning, Performance Assessment, and Common Core
Standards*, Bob Lenz, Justin Wells and Sally Kingston document their work at Envision Schools. Published in 2015, they
claim the following about the Envision Schools program:

*Case studies on our schools, published by Stanford
University researchers, found that Envision Schools graduates are entering and persisting in college at rates far ahead
of their demographically comparable peers. One hundred*

---

98   Jal Mehta and Sarah Fine, "Opinion | High School Doesn't Have to Be
     Boring," *The New York Times*, March 30, 2019, sec. Opinion, https://
     www.nytimes.com/2019/03/30/opinion/sunday/fix-high-school-ed-
     ucation.html.

percent of African American and Latino 2012 graduates completed the courses required for University of California/ California State University eligibility at Impact Academy, an Envision school.[99]

What is crucial about the philosophy shared in this book is their emphasis on depth; this is something that, as a systems thinker, I jump up and down applauding when I read it.

Citing how technology has exponentially increased the amount of information available to every individual, they profess a particular view of how best to proceed:

> *. . . the answer to exploding knowledge is not more schooling but a different kind of schooling. This is what the concept of deeper learning is all about and why it came to be. To pretend that we can "cover" everything that students need to know is to tilt at windmills. We must rid ourselves of any residual notions that education is the transmission of needed knowledge. Rather, we are teaching skills, and one skill most generally: how to ride a tsunami of knowledge whose future content we can't even begin to imagine. . . when deep, conceptual understanding is attained, learning is enduring, flexible, and real.*[100]

---

99 Bob Lenz, Justin Wells, and Sally Kingston, *Transforming Schools Using Project-Based Learning, Performance Assessment, and Common Core Standards* (London: John Wiley & Sons, 2015), 3.

100 Ibid., 9.

It requires a flexible mind to simply entertain the thought that the purpose of school is *not* to "[transmit] needed knowledge." Instead, the purpose is or should be to equip students with the capacity to handle "a tsunami of knowledge" skillfully and for real. The capacity for wisdom and discernment arises from this more in-depth level of education discussed, and not "transmission of needed knowledge." Likewise, the author's emphasis on creativity and the student's capacity to create is also far more important than we will sufficiently attend to here.

Incidentally, Bob Lenz is CEO of the Buck Institute for Education, located right here in Novato. You can learn more about what resources are available on their website pblworks. org. (PBL stands for Project Based Learning.)

How do we meet UN SDG #4 Quality Education for everyone? Through vastly improved, fairer, and friendly school funding policies at the local level, including district consolidation. Through high quality project-based learning. And through granting a much greater sense of personhood to children and youth than has often been afforded them in the past. If generation upon generation of school attendees complain of being "bored," then there isn't something wrong with the kids, there's something wrong with the schools and the society that allows this state to continue.

– CHAPTER 5 –

SDG #5 Gender Equality

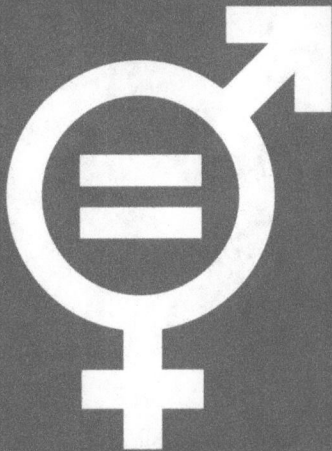

Where are we?

According to Paul Hawken, editor of *Drawdown: The Most Comprehensive Plan Ever Proposed to Reverse Global Warming*, "The number one solution to reversing global warming is empowering girls and women."[101] "Empowering" in this context he defines as two areas equally: access to quality education through secondary school, and access to comprehensive family planning. Hawken and the Drawdown findings are echoing decades of work done previously that document the positive, systemic power of societies allowing girls and women these same basic human rights of education and family planning.

The book *What Works in Girls' Education: Evidence for the World's Best Investment*, provides data to support this claim. The publisher, the Brookings Institute, lists these areas of benefit:

- Better outcomes in economic areas of growth and incomes
- Reduced rates of infant and maternal mortality
- Reduced rates of child marriage
- Reduced rates of the incidence of HIV/AIDS and malaria

---

101 talkingsticktv, "Paul Hawken - Drawdown: The Most Comprehensive Plan Ever Proposed to Reverse Global Warming," YouTube, April 25, 2017, https://www.youtube.com/watch?v=0zaTGMl11hs.

- Increased agricultural productivity
- Increased resilience to natural disasters
- Women's empowerment

We can add to this list reversing global warming, and a number of additional social and ecological benefits. Download the 338-page book for free at brookings.edu.

You would think, given the known and well-documented positive power of empowering women and girls that it would be perhaps *the* top policy and social priority of all nations. This is not what we have seen in the world, nor in our own country. In this chapter we spend extra time laying a broader context for the topic of gender equality, specifically with regard to a group that is particularly negatively targeted, Native North American women.

Gender Equality in the United States

It's challenging to think about gender equality in the United States in the wake of the June 24, 2022 Supreme Court decision to overturn Roe v. Wade and the right to an abortion. As we will see, we are doing well on some gender equality topics in the United States and perhaps Marin in particular. But some aspects of gender equality seem to be perennially stuck in place.

In a list of countries ranked from best to worst for gender equality by worldpopulationreview.com, the United States is number 30 among 155 countries.[102] The measure takes into

---

102 "Gender Equality by Country," World Population Review, 2021, https://worldpopulationreview.com/country-rankings/gender-equality-by-country.

consideration economic opportunity, educational, health and political access.

As you can imagine, gender inequality has many real-world manifestations. With regard to economic manifestations, one impact is access to purchasing a home. A study published in 2022 by the real estate sales website Zillow claims that nationally, if gaps in pay between men and women were closed, women could afford to purchase 18% more of the housing market than they can at present.[103] Happily, they also confirm that the gap is shrinking, though, more so in certain geographies and job sectors than others.

Equal Pay Day

This date is set as an annual observation of the day on which women's earnings match men's earnings nationally from the year before. In 2022, Equal Pay Day was March 15th. Thus, statistically speaking, a woman would need to work all of 2021 plus two-and-a-half months into 2022 to match the annual income of a man. In other words, women on average earn $0.83 cents for every $1.00 a man earns. As you can see from the quoted facts below on the AAUW.org website (American Association of University Women), this date is much further out for different groups of women:

Asian American, Native Hawaiian and Pacific Islander Women's Equal Pay Day is May 3. Asian American and

---

103 Nichole Bachaud, "Domino Effect: Gender Pay Gap Has Implications for Women Home Buyers," Zillow Research, March 30, 2022, https://www.zillow.com/research/equal-pay-day-2022-30887/.

Pacific Islander women are paid 75 cents for every dollar paid to White men.

LGBTQIA+ Equal Pay Awareness Day is June 15. Without enough data to make calculations, this day raises awareness about the wage gap experienced by LGBTQIA+ folks.

Moms' Equal Pay Day is September 8. Moms are paid 58 cents for every dollar paid to dads.

Black Women's Equal Pay Day is September 21. Black women are paid 58 cents for every dollar paid to White men.

Native Women's Equal Pay Day is November 30. Native women are paid 50 cents for every dollar paid to White men.

Latina's Equal Pay Day is December 8. Latinas are paid 49 cents for every dollar paid to White men.[104]

Let's just pause for a moment and acknowledge that, at the extreme end of the spectrum, the value placed on the labor of Native American and Latina women is about half of the value placed on the labor of White men. And according to the data quoted above, none of the other groups cited are doing a whole lot better. Donella Meadows brings the harsh reality of economic differences into sharp focus: "Money measures

104 "Equal Pay Day Calendar," American Association of University Women, accessed August 26, 2022, https://www.aauw.org/resources/article/equal-pay-day-calendar/.

something real and has real meaning, therefore, people who are paid less are literally worth less."[105] This is not the reality we want to be living, nor the reality we want future generations to inherit.

Gender Equality & Native Americans

I don't want to generalize too much about the equality or inequality of men and women in every Native North American group. Nevertheless, there is a reasonable amount of documentation that these cultures historically had gender roles that were far and away more equitable than those of European societies, and in some cases have managed to hang on to greater equality despite colonialism, acculturation, and the impact of poverty and other extreme challenges issuing from these forces.

This section has two goals. One is to attend in greater depth to a topic specific to Native North Americans, who, as noted earlier, are often overlooked. The other is that it allows us to gain a contrasting view of how gender equality may look in another culture; to somewhat dismantle the seeming inevitability of male dominance, given how long it has lasted in European cultures.

Kathleen A. Ward quotes Chief Sitting Bull to provide context for the historical transition from tribal life and relative gender equality to colonially-influenced inequality:

---

105 Donella Meadows, *Thinking in Systems: A Primer* (New York: Chelsea Green Publishing, 2008), 163.

Tribal leaders resisted these forced cultural alterations, but their pleas unfortunately fell on deaf ears. The powerful Sioux Chief, Sitting Bull, said, "take pity on my women. . . . The young men can be like the White men, can till the soil, supply the food and clothing. They will take the work out of the hands of women. And the women . . . will be stripped of all which gave them power." Sitting Bull's statements reflected the attitude of many Indians that by adopting Western values and customs power was being taken away from native women, and they were being sentenced to a life of persecution and abuse.[106]

One might add, "sentenced to a life of persecution and abuse," much like the situation faced by *White* women in North America (and many parts of the world) across the centuries. Another article, this one posted to the National Park Service website, underscores this basic pattern:

Rape and other acts of violence against women by most accounts were rare in Indigenous societies prior to European contact and dealt with harshly in the rare event they occurred. White women who spent time on Native American reservations routinely commented on the degree of safety they felt and the freedom to move at their own will and discretion. A mail carrier in the late 1800's told a New York Herald reporter visiting the Seneca nation,

106 Kathleen A. Ward, "Before and after the White Man: Indian Women, Property, Progress, and Power," *Connecticut Public Interest Law Journal* 6 (2006): 267.

"A White woman can go around alone among them or on the most desolate roads with perfect safety. I'd rather have my wife or daughter go around alone at night in this reservation than in the town I live in." A schoolteacher concurred: "It is the only place at which I ever taught in which I never was insulted, . . . I've heard the same from every woman teacher I know on the reservation."[107]

One should not extrapolate these comments to mean that every North American tribal group had perfect gender equality. Doing so would put us in the typical grove of idealizing or romanticizing indigenous peoples. But nor should we ignore testimonials that paint a picture of important cultural differences between indigenous groups and Europeans.

Two-Spirit

In some Native North American groups greater equality extended to gender diverse individuals and cultural practices as well. According to the Indian Health Service, the phrase "Two-Spirit" refers to a great variety of forms that differ across tribes and individuals. So too was this social fluidity and flexibility violently diminished by the arrival of Europeans:

The disruptions caused by conquest and disease, together with the efforts of missionaries, government agents,

---

107 Sally Wagner, "How Native American Women Inspired the Women's Rights Movement," National Park Service, April 15, 2020, https://www.nps.gov/articles/000/how-native-american-women-inspired-the-women-s-rights-movement.htm.

boarding schools, and White settlers resulted in the loss of many traditions in Native communities. Two-spirit roles, in particular, were singled out for condemnation, interference, and many times violence. As a result, two-spirit traditions and practices went underground or disappeared in many tribes.[108]

Missing and Murdered Indigenous Women
It's a troubling fact that today's Native Americans, in particular women, have some of the lowest quality of life outcomes of any group. Indigenous females and African American females together share many of the worst statistics. As cited above, Native American women and Latina women are on average economically valued least in comparison to White males.

You may be familiar with the acronym "MMIW," which stands for Missing and Murdered Indigenous Women. The prevalence of Indigenous women and girls being abducted, raped and killed is dramatically disproportionate to the population at large, though, due to myriad factors, data about those who go missing or who are attacked or murdered is often full of holes or missing entirely. As the authors of an article on the National Indigenous Women's Resource Center (NIWRC) website states,

A person's relationship to a problem often reflects their framework or worldview for understanding it. While

---

108 "Two Spirit," Indian Health Service, accessed August 26, 2022, https://www.ihs.gov/lgbt/health/twospirit/.

violence against Native women is committed by individuals—abusers, rapists, traffickers—it is federal colonial policies and laws that created the social setting for such crimes. While living in the same country the worldview of the colonized versus that of the colonizer are fundamentally distinct.[109]

This is an important point. There is a long and dark history between Native North Americans and European colonizers of North America; a historical context that influences both the way our society responds to the abduction, rape and murder of Indigenous girls and women, as well as the fact of the prevalence of the attacks in the first place. In short, our society collectively has put Native women and girls in an especially vulnerable position. From this same source:

The shift from international diplomacy to federal colonialism undermined the right of Indian Nations to self-government and the authority to protect Native women. Current federal Indian law is often referred to as a maze of injustice. It lacks logic and a moral standard because it was created based on the drive of the United States to lay stake to Tribal lands and resources.

---

109 "MMIW: Understanding the Missing and Murdered Indigenous Women Crisis Beyond Individual Acts of Violence," NIWRC, June 2020, https://www.niwrc.org/restoration-magazine/june-2020/mmiw-understanding-missing-and-murdered-indigenous-women-crisis.

In short, the *purpose* of federal Indian law is not justice. This body of law was originally intended to maintain *power over*. That makes human beings themselves expendable; tangential to the goal itself. An article from *National Geographic* about missing and murdered Native women in California makes a salient point in this vein:

> *Abby Abinanti, chief judge of the Yurok Tribal Court in Klamath...addresses the lack of trust more bluntly. "The Yurok word for policemen translates to 'men who steal children,'" she says. "The first time we ever met them was when they came and stole children as indentured slaves or for the boarding schools. So, you have a natural resistance on our part."[110]*

The authors of the NIWRC article go on to say the following:

> *The crisis of MMIW is a national crime pattern. The complete storyboard for this crime pattern is not two individuals and a crime scene but all of the above--the government, culture, and economics--layered upon the lives of Native women and Indian nations. Understanding the legal and social infrastructure that place Native women in harm's way are essential to changing this crime story of the last 500 years.*

---

110 Brandi Morin, "Picturesque California Conceals a Crisis of Missing Indigenous Women," History, March 15, 2022, https://www.nationalgeographic.com/history/article/california-crisis-missing-indigenous-women.

We can see that the position of Native women and Indian nations in the context of European-dominated society is an extreme shade of a European cultural norm that prioritizes masculinity and males over femininity and females, and often pits them against one another. It's no wonder that both gender diversity and gender equality are a threat to this ridged cultural background.

Gender Equality & Gender Diversity

As quoted above, Equal Pay Day for LGBTQIA+ (which as of this writing stands for Lesbian, Gay, Bisexual, Transgender, Queer, Intersex, Asexual, plus acknowledgment of variations with the plus sign) is June 15th. This is a strictly symbolic date due to limited data about this diverse group.

An important point to understanding gender diversity is to learn how people who identify with the LGBTQIA+ category differentiate between the terms "sex" and "gender." Sam Killermann, comedian and social justice activist, provides an entertaining and helpful "Genderbread Person" infographic on his website genderbread.org, which he characterizes as, "A teaching tool for breaking the big concept of gender down into bite-sized, digestible pieces." He provides four terms:

Anatomical Sex: Sex (sometimes called biological sex, anatomical sex, or physical sex) is comprised of things like genitals, chromosomes, hormones, body hair, and more. But one thing it's not: gender.

Gender Identity: Your psychological sense of self. Who you, in your head, know yourself to be, based on how much you align (or don't align) with what you understand to be the options for gender.

Gender Expression: The ways you present gender, through your actions, clothing, demeanor, and more. Your out-ward-facing self, and how that's interpreted by others based on gender norms.

Attraction: Like sex, attraction isn't really a component of gender. However, we often conflate sexual orientation with gender, or categorize the attraction we experience in gendered ways.[111]

Just as law enforcement and other government entities have done a poor job of collecting and reporting ethnicity and other important details relating to attacks against Indigenous women, the 2017 National Crime Victimization Survey was actually the first "comprehensive criminal victimization data to include information on the sexual orientation and gender identity of respondents."[112] The report documented that in that year,

---

111 "Genderbread Person v4.0," The Genderbread Person, 0, accessed August 26, 2022, https://www.genderbread.org/.
112 "LGBT People Nearly Four Times More Likely Than Non-Lgbt People to Be Victims of Violent Crime," Williams Institute, October 2, 2020, https://williamsinstitute.law.ucla.edu/press/ncvs-lgbt-violence-press-release/.

. . . LGBT people experienced 71.1 victimizations per 1,000 people, compared to 19.2 victimizations per 1,000 people for non-LGBT people. LGBT people had higher rates of serious violence victimization in almost every type of violent crime. . .

Data from the 2019 Youth Risk Behavior Survey (YRBS) document significantly higher rates of bullying at U.S. high schools for LGBTQIA+ people.[113] Youth who identify with this group reported "not going to school because of safety concerns" at a much higher rate than students outside of this group; 13.5% and 7.5% respectively.

For more insight into the issues surrounding LGBTQIA+ groups, refer to sdgmarin.org/gender-equality and the May 15, 2021 event hosted by UNA Marin featuring Pri Bertucci, CEO of [DIVERSITY BBOX].

Gender Equality in California

According to a 2022 Mercury News article, "LGBTQ students may be the most bullied of all student groups in California."[114] The article cites data gathered by the 2019 National School Climate Survey who reported "that California schools were

---

113 Assistant Secretary for Public Affairs (ASPA), "LGBTQI+ Youth," Text, Stop Bullying, September 24, 2019, https://www.stopbullying. gov/bullying/lgbtq.

114 Beau Yarbough, "How California Students from Marginalized Groups Are Working to Stop Bullying," *The Sun*, March 24, 2022, https://www.sbsun.com/2022/03/24/marginalized-students-in-california-face-higher-levels-of-bullying.

not safe for most lesbian, gay, bisexual, transgender, and queer (LGBTQ) secondary school students."[115]

Again, this collective challenge with gender, sexuality and identity is rooted in the larger picture of valuing males above females, masculinity above femineity, and overall, the strongest and largest individuals and groups over the weaker, smaller individuals and groups. There are important questions we will not explore here about the cultural and religious mores that inform and reinforce gender inequality, as well as the socioeconomic factors that exacerbate the situation in a given context. Our society's lack of rights of passage and meaningful ritual that help individuals to develop a strong sense of self and agency also relate strongly to gender equality.

California Compared to Other States

The website WalletHub published an article in 2021 that provides a look at all 50 states ranked on 17 weighted indicators across three areas of gender equality: "1) Workplace Environment, 2) Education & Health and 3) Political Empowerment".[116] California scored #6, with Iowa the next highest (in particular due to having the second smallest income gap). Nevada ranks #1, notably with the "Smallest Work Hours Gap" and "Smallest Political Representation Gap" of all 50 states.

115 "School Climate for LGBTQ Students in California" (California: GLSEN, 2019), https://www.glsen.org/sites/default/files/2021-01/California-Snapshot-2019.pdf.

116 Adam McCann, "2022's Best & Worst States for Women's Equality," Wallet Hub, August 22, 2022, https://wallethub.com/edu/best-and-worst-states-for-women-equality/5835.

Nevertheless, out of a possible perfect score of 100, Nevada's cumulative total is just 77.55. Therefore, the highest performing state in the nation for gender equality earns a C+. California is next to failing, with the equivalent of a D+ considering our 67.01 score out of 100.

Gender Equality in Marin County

Gender equality here in Marin County cannot reasonably be expected to differ in any significant way from our larger social context. However, the acute wealth gap in Marin can and does exacerbate some of the issues faced by women. In an April 2022 article, Vicki Larson, reporter for the Marin Independent Journal, published an article titled, "Being a woman in Marin is tougher than ever."[117] She cites her own experience as well as that of fellow Marin residents.

Women and Poverty in Marin

We discussed the problems with the federal poverty line measure earlier. Nevertheless, Census data of course references the federal poverty line heavily. Data cited on datausa.io summarize poverty by age and sex.[118] It shows that in nearly all of their 13 age categories, females live in poverty at greater rates than males. Altogether, females experience poverty at a rate 15%

---

117 Vicki Larson, "Vicki Larson: Being a Woman in Marin Is Tougher than Ever," *Marin Independent Journal*, April 25, 2022, https://www.marinij.com/2022/04/25/vicki-larson-being-a-woman-in-marin-is-tougher-than-ever/.

118 "Marin County, Ca," Data USA, 2020, https://datausa.io/profile/geo/marin-county-ca.

higher than males in Marin. Programs such as the YWCA 50+ Employment Support Program provide job training and related services for women in this demographic, citing the age and gender discrimination in the job market that afflicts older women in particular.

Women and Income in Marin
With regard to wages by sex, datausa.io reports the average salary for a male in California at $81,539, and $64,688 for females in 2019, a nearly $17,000 difference. We can reasonably assume that the average salary difference between men and women in Marin is similar to that of California overall. This means that the average woman in Marin earns approximately 20% less than that of the average man.

Intimate Partner Violence & Domestic Violence
Strictly speaking, these two terms are quite close but not precisely the same in their meaning. While "Intimate Partner Violence" (IPV) is used to refer to violence between two people in a relationship, whether or not they live together, "Domestic Violence" can happen between any two people in a household.[119] However, given the prevalence of the term "Domestic Violence," and the relatively new term IPV, they are often used interchangeably.

---

119 "The Language We Use," Women Against Abuse, accessed December 1, 2022, https://www.womenagainstabuse.org/education-resources/the-language-we-use.

The Center for Domestic Peace in San Rafael cites domestic violence as the number one violent crime in Marin County.[120] They say on their website, "Since our founding in 1977, we have responded to the needs of more than 195,000 women and children affected by domestic violence, as well as more than 29,000 men who have been violent."

Domestic violence or Intimate Partner Violence is not a private affair. The impacts ripple thought the lives of the victims, witnesses (frequently, children) and thus, the community. For example,

Significantly more U.S. women and men with a history of contact sexual violence or stalking by any perpetrator, or physical violence by an intimate partner, reported asthma, irritable bowel syndrome, frequent headaches, chronic pain, difficulty sleeping, and limitations in their activities compared to women and men without a history of these forms of violence. More U.S. women and men reporting these forms of violence also consider their physical and mental health to be poor compared to non-victims.[121]

This same report states that nationally, "1 in 4 women (26.4%) and 1 in 9 men (11.0%) have experienced contact

---

120 Marla H, "About Us," Center for Domestic Peace, accessed August 27, 2022, https://centerfordomesticpeace.org/about-us/.

121 S.G. Smith et al., "The National Intimate Partner and Sexual Violence Survey (NISVS)" (National Center for Injury Prevention and Control, Centers for Disease Control and Prevention, 2017), 18, https://www.cdc.gov/violenceprevention/pdf/NISVS-StateReportBook.pdf.

sexual violence, physical violence, and/or stalking by an intimate partner in their lifetime and reported an IPV-related impact (injury, fear, concern for safety, needing services)."[122] KidsData.org reports that the economic cost of Intimate Partner Violence is $8.3 billion annually, and $3.6 trillion over the lifetimes of those involved.

If you or someone you know is or may be suffering from this type of violence, the Center for Domestic Peace offers a help line for domestic abuse support, (415)924-6616.

Human Trafficking
Human trafficking is another insidious issue in Marin, and there are organizations working to prevent harm and offer support to victims. The Marin Coalition to End Human Trafficking is a partnership of various local government agencies and NGOs aiming to both increase awareness of human trafficking—including both sex trafficking and labor trafficking—and get help for victims. Speak Safe – Save Adolescents from Exploitation focuses on educating youth in Marin to know what to look for with regard to exploitation of Marin youth.

According to worldpopulationreview.com, the United States is one of the worst countries for human trafficking: "It is estimated that 199,000 incidents occur within the United States every year," though only 11,500 cases were reported.[123]

---

122 Ibid., 16.
123 "Human Trafficking Statistics by State 2022," World Population Review, 2022, https://worldpopulationreview.com/state-rankings/human-trafficking-statistics-by-state.

While California is reported to have the highest total number of human trafficking cases annually, it is listed as #7 on a per 100k person basis, with Nevada ranked first.[124]

Finally, the Marin County Civil Grand Jury published a report in 2016 citing that, according to the FBI, San Francisco is one of the thirteen highest human sex trafficking areas nationwide; a distinction that also includes Los Angeles and San Diego.[125] In short:

Human sex trafficking is hidden, but thriving in Marin because it is:

Next door to San Francisco, one of the nation's top hubs for human sex trafficking, making it an easy stop on the "circuit" of victims transported around the Bay area and region.

Home to many wealthy "johns" able to pay with cash, thus enabling traffickers to charge more.

Geographically desirable to traffickers since it is near a major highway (101).[126]

The report notes that victims come from all socioeconomic groups, and about 30% are children, saying,

124 Ibid.

125 "Marin's Hidden Human Sex Trafficking Challenge: It's Happening In Our Backyard" (Marin County Civil Grand Jury, June 16, 2016), https://www.marincounty.org/~/media/files/departments/gj/reports-responses/2015/marin-hidden-human-sex-trafficking-challenge.pdf?la=en.

126 Ibid.

Children in higher income bracket families are vulnerable as they often spend more time alone and generally live in households with fewer family members. As a result, access to unmonitored computer use often increases, bringing with it the risk of unsafe communications.

Finally, the report cites labor trafficking as well, saying,

Representatives from two victim advocate organizations interviewed said that they had received reports of labor trafficking for nursing homes, ranching, and farming, with one citing a victim rescued from forced labor as a nanny.

To review the "Where are we?" portion of this chapter, as with most of the other SDGs, Marin County has both some unique advantages and disadvantages when it comes to SDG #5 Gender Equality. Overall, however, we average out to about the same level as the rest of the state and the nation: we are making incremental improvements, but we are still a significant distance from equality. Thus, we would have to work creatively and diligently to create local conditions that sustainably foster genuine gender equality.

Where do we want to get to?

First, a bit of good news. To recap, worldpopulationreview.com measures gender equality based on economic opportunity, education, health, and political access. The Public Policy Institute of California ranks Marin County as having the highest average educational attainment of all California counties, with 60% of the population over 25 possessing at least a bachelor's degree.[127] Statisticalatlas.com provides data in their "Educational Attainment Sex Ratio" that women in Marin County who are 25 years or older are a few percentage points *more* likely than men to have a degree beyond a high school diploma (61.2% for males versus 65.2% for females).[128] (It is unclear what years statisticalatlas.com is drawing their data from.)

Also, if you look at the elected officials in Marin County, males and females are very close in terms of representation in political office. This is in contrast to the global picture. According to the United Nations, in Europe and North America women only occupy about 35% of "local deliberative bodies."[129]

The Institute for Health Metrics and Evaluation (IHME) provides a snapshot of life expectancy for males and females in all counties of the United States. In keeping with larger trends,[130]

---

127 Cesar Perez, Hans Johnson, and Vicki Hsieh, "Geography of Educational Attainment in California," Public Policy Institute of California, April 6, 2021, https://www.ppic.org/blog/geography-of-educational-attainment-in-california/.

128 "The Demographic Statistical Atlas of the United States," Statistics Atlas, accessed August 27, 2022, https://statisticalatlas.com/county/California/Marin-County/Educational-Attainment.

129 "Facts and Figures: Women's Leadership and Political Participation," UN Women, January 15, 2021, https://www.unwomen.org/en/what-we-do/leadership-and-political-participation/facts-and-figures.

130 "Around the Globe, Women Outlive Men," Population Reference Bureau, September 1, 2001, https://www.prb.org/resources/around-the-globe-women-outlive-men/.

females tend to outlive men in Marin County by about three years.[131]

In other words, in three of the four areas defining gender equality—educational attainment, health, and political representation—Marin's gender equality looks pretty good. This analysis leaves out differences in educational attainment between, say, African American females and White males. This way of measuring gender equality also leaves out language barriers and concerns over immigration status that may lead Latina women to not seek reproductive services, though the overwhelming majority support providing women with access.[132] Still, it is crucial that we acknowledge where we are doing well: so-called "bright spots" where things are heading in the right direction—toward great gender equality—need further attention and support.

The obvious, stark differences between male and female equality in Marin, however, is in the realm of economics. Going back to the source cited above, Statisticalatlas.com shows that when you look at "Median Earnings by Educational Attainment," in all degree attainment categories men out-earn women (see Figure 16).[133]

131 "County Profile: Marin County, California," Health Data, 2016, https://www.healthdata.org/sites/default/files/files/county_profiles/US/2015/County_Report_Marin_County_California.pdf.

132 "Latina/O Voters' Views and Experiences Around Reproductive Health" (Latina Institute, October 4, 2018), https://www.latinainstitute.org/sites/default/files/NLIRH%20Survey%20Report_F_0.pdf.

133 "Educational Attainment in Marin County, California," Statistical Atlas, August 28, 2022, https://statisticalatlas.com/county/California/Marin-County/Educational-Attainment#figure/educational-attainment-sex-ratio.

Median Earnings by Educational Attainment [#11]

By sex among population 25 years old and over with earnings.
Scope: population of California and Marin County

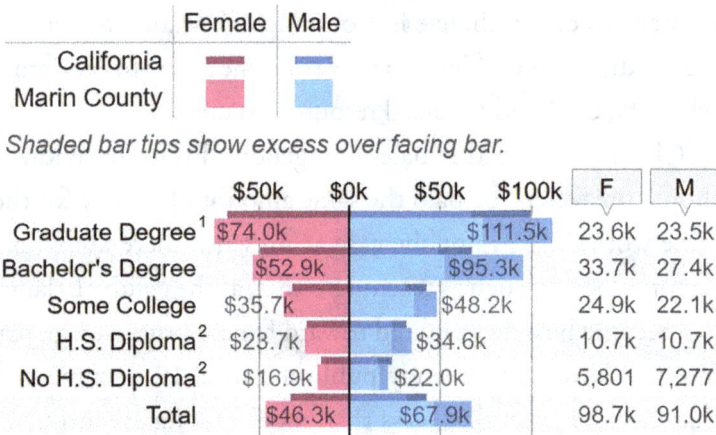

	Female	Male
California	—	—
Marin County	▮	▮

Shaded bar tips show excess over facing bar.

	$50k $0k $50k $100k	F	M
Graduate Degree[1]	$74.0k $111.5k	23.6k	23.5k
Bachelor's Degree	$52.9k $95.3k	33.7k	27.4k
Some College	$35.7k $48.2k	24.9k	22.1k
H.S. Diploma[2]	$23.7k $34.6k	10.7k	10.7k
No H.S. Diploma[2]	$16.9k $22.0k	5,801	7,277
Total	$46.3k $67.9k	98.7k	91.0k

F females with given highest level of educational attainment
M males with given highest level of educational attainment
[1] or professional degree   [2] H.S. = High School

Figure 16 - Marin County and CA, Unknown Year(s), from statisticalatlas.com

For example, for individuals who did not earn a high school diploma, the median earnings cited (based on US Census Bureau and the 2012 – 2016 American Community Survey) were $16,900 per year for women, and $22,000 per year for men (a 23%, or $5,100 annual difference). At the other end of the educational attainment scale, there is a slightly greater disparity, with women who hold a graduate degree having median earnings of $74,000, and men showing median earnings of $111,500 (a 33%, or $37,500 annual difference). (The "F" and "M" columns on the far right indicate the number of "Females" and "Males" whose educational attainment was included in the date for that line.)

Again, if we are looking at economic opportunity, education, health and political access, the main category in which we want to create change is economic. We want women and gender diverse individuals to have the same access to economic self-sufficiency and financial resources as men.

Clearly males and females and gender diverse individuals should on average be paid the same amount of money for the same work. This is not the case at present. There are whole sectors of jobs—such as teaching—that, as the gender balance has become heavily weighted toward females, the average pay has gone down.[134] A study published in 2019 documented that "women earn 8.9% less than men" among executives at nonprofit organizations.[135] At the local level, we want local organizations to take responsibility for ensuring equal pay for equal work between males and females.

Further, given the dramatic differences that arise when comparing the incomes of White men and Latina women, as in the Equal Pay Day statistics we reviewed above, Marin County would need to find a way to support Latina and other non-White women in strong and unique ways that go against the tide of the wider society.

134 Elizabeth Boyle, "The Feminization of Teaching in America" (Massachusetts Institute of Technology, 2004), https://stuff.mit.edu/afs/athena.mit.edu/org/w/wgs/prize/eb04.html.
135 Niki Gianakaris, "Gender Pay Gaps in Nonprofits Are Even Greater When There Is Room for Salary Negotiations," Drexel, May 4, 2021, http://drexel.edu/news/archive/2021/May/Study-on-gender-pay-gaps-at-nonprofits.

But again, supporting, say, a 50-year-old African American woman to attain higher levels of education only to situate her in a job market that more highly values (as reflected by average pay) the labor of men over that of women—over non-White women and/or older women in particular—is not a full answer either.

Wealthy Women & the 1%

Before we look at how to ameliorate our local gender inequality, we need to factor in an important, often overlooked demographic we have here in Marin that is hiding in plain sight.

In the Forbes 2022 list of the 20 richest people in the world, only two are women.[136] Though this group is at the extreme end of the spectrum, their gender inequality refracts down into the rest of the global population. The inequality seems to diminish in size the closer to the middle class you look. As we have seen looking at averages, however, the economic inequality—and the presence of domestic violence against women—is still very much in this group as well.

An article on contexts.org, "Gender in the One Percent," documents that the source of wealthy family's income is predominantly from the male's side.[137] They go on to profile the resulting influence of males and females both within their households and in their larger communities.

---

136 Richard Mille, "The Richest People In The World," Forbes, accessed August 27, 2022, https://www.forbes.com/billionaires/.

137 Jill E. Yavorsky, Lisa A. Keister, and Yue Qian, "Gender in the One Percent," *Contexts* 19, no. 1 (February 1, 2020): 12–17, https://doi.org/10.1177/1536504220902196.

The authors state the following:

In this piece, we discuss gender income dynamics in the one percent and show that White, heterosexual, married men earn most of the income in this elite group. We propose that, as a result of their disproportionate contribution to household income, men in the one percent likely exercise considerable power, both inside and outside of the household.

This article, published March 15, 2020, qualifies membership in the "one percent" demographic as a household that has an annual income of $845,000 or greater. But the gender differences are stark. They state, ". . . 85% of one percent households do not depend on women's income to be in this elite group." And for women who are in this group based on their own income, about a quarter of them are married to men whose own income also qualifies. Conversely, "men have more disparate spousal incomes than women and marry a high-income woman only 3% of the time." While there are internal, household power differences that issue from this gender-based income disparity, that is perhaps just the tip of the proverbial iceberg:

Women in one percent households, whose income is largely not responsible for the household's elite status and who in many cases are not employed, likely have significantly less authority over the direction of political campaign contributions and do not have the same high-powered connections or influence as their breadwinning husbands.[138]

The authors of this article take pains to state that they are not trying to paint women in elite households as victims:

To be clear, we are not claiming that (mostly White, heterosexual, married) women in the one percent are disenfranchised; rather, we suggest that a small group of homogenous men likely hold most of the substantive status and influence in the one percent. This phenomenon may have important social and political implications.

They explain that other research has documented the prevalence of money from wealthy men in the pockets of politicians, and that the politics of wealthy men and the policies enacted by politicians are generally more conservative than the politics of the general population, male or female. This leads to elected officials tending to be more conservative overall than the general population.

Thus, we see the larger implications for society as a whole directly linked to the power dynamics in individual households. This is a complex set of factors that takes careful study to map out, as well as a willingness to look in greater detail at the personal income levels of higher income households. For example, perhaps the U.S. Census categories that range from "Less than $10,000" annually to "$200,000 or more" are

---

138 Ibid.

not granular enough? Dealing with wealth and income as a community is nearly as confronting as dealing with domestic abuse, and the two can be interlinked.

Domestic Abuse in Wealthy Households

Referencing the note made in the introduction about wealth not equaling well-being, domestic abuse in wealthy families is uniquely under-reported and challenging to document, due to the privacy barriers wealth enables. The social factors at work in preventing women (or men for that matter) and the children of wealthy parents from reporting abuse are extreme and hard to fathom.

The 2001 book *Not To People Like Us: Hidden Abuse In Upscale Marriages*, is one of very few that deal with gender power issues in wealthy families. (*The Golden Ghetto*, mentioned earlier, is another resource.) In particular, the author, a psychotherapist, discusses her experience with clients who are well-educated, successful women stuck in abusive marriages.

While the reviews of this book are full of personal statements by women sharing their own experiences of this phenomena, as well as repeated notes about the lack of attention it receives, Amazon's related book suggestions at the bottom of the page don't provide a single additional book for wealthy women experiencing abuse.

A woman with low or no income may suffer from a lack of resources to escape a violent relationship. It would seem that a woman in a wealthy household would have much greater resources at her disposal. But she may be in a uniquely challenging situation issuing from her well-resourced partner removing her access to money, and potentially intimidating her through hired lawyers, private investigators, or thugs.

How do we get there?

SDG #5 Gender Equality is, as we have reviewed, the Global Goal that we in Marin County are closest to reaching. And yet, the larger economic and social forces that prevent true gender equality are tricky, to say the least. Inequality runs deep in our culture, whether between men and women, or between gender diverse and "cisgender" individuals. ("Cis" by the way is Latin for "on the near side of." It refers to individuals who identify as their sex assigned at birth.)

We make a mistake when we think that achieving gender equality for all is merely about making the world a nicer place. Our civilization is living out at a profound level the problems that gender imbalance bring.

In addition to the political implications noted above, consider this example. The original electric car market was marketed to women; they were at least somewhat preferred by women as an alternative to the louder, smellier gasoline cars that you had to crank to start.[139] Maybe if we had greater gender equality in the first half of the 20th century, we would not have lost the widespread use of the electric car as we did?

---

139 Virginia Scharff, "Femininity and the Electric Car: Early Automobiles and 'Separate Spheres,'" in *Early Automobiles and "Separate Spheres"* (New York: Free Press, 1991), http://www.autolife.umd.umich.edu/ Gender/Scharff/G_casestudy1.htm.

Warren Wells of the Marin County Bicycle Coalition, at a
UNA Marin event in 2022, explained that data shows repeatedly that women don't bike as frequently as men in our area
(and many others) due to safety concerns.[140] A quote from an
article articulates the situation:

> *There is a big gender gap in cycling worldwide, due largely
> to greater safety concerns on the part of women. In coun-
> tries where cycling comprises a large percentage of overall
> trips (greater than 25% mode share), researchers have
> found gender parity in bicycle use—indeed, women in the
> Netherlands bike more often than men. In contrast, in the
> United States, men and women are equally likely to walk
> to their destination, yet men are three times as likely to
> ride a bicycle.[141]*

The authors summarize how this situation equates to gender equality:

> *When cities fail to invest in cycling transportation infra-
> structure—bicycle lanes physically separated from traffic,
> reduced road speeds, safety improvements to intersections,*

140 United Nations Association - Marin County Chapter, "SDG 11
    Sustainable Cities & Communities Marin County California - UNA
    Marin Chapter," YouTube, May 22, 2022, https://www.youtube.com/
    watch?v=AtzaQpUHNo0.
141 Paul Steinberg, "Women Bike Less, But Do They Voice More HSA
    Blog," Harvey Mudd collage, November 16, 2020, https://www.
    hmc.edu/hsa/2020/11/16/women-bike-less-but-do-they-voice-
    more-by-paul-steinberg/.

better lighting and other measures—women have less options for exercise and recreation, and fewer alternatives for commuting to work and for completing household chores. Car-dependent cities impose an indirect cost on women as well because women bear the primary responsibility for chauffeuring family members who cannot drive.

There are no two ways about it: Marin County is a car-dependent place. It's reasonable to assume that anywhere between 25% and 50% of people in our county don't actually drive, either because they are too young, elderly, physically unable to drive, choose not to drive, or simply don't have access to a vehicle. This quote points out that it's the women in the family who are most typically the ones who try to fill the gap, carting everyone else around.

SDG Cross-Talk

We can conclude from this complex set of factors that reliable, safe, affordable public transportation, along with an abundance of safe walking and biking paths, are a matter of gender equality. Therefore, one way of moving us closer to achieving SDG #5 Gender Equality is a solution that not only better meets the needs of women and families but is also better for overall human health (in terms of exercise biking and walking) and the health of the environment (in terms of reducing carbon emissions and the embedded energy and materials cost of manufacturing individual automobiles).

In fact, if you look at the SDGs we have covered so far—#1 No Poverty, #2 Zero Hunger, #3 Good Health and

Well-Being, and #4 Quality Education—a pattern starts to emerge. Achieving #5 Gender Equality is inextricably woven into each of these Global Goals.

SDG #1 No Poverty and SDG #5 Gender Equality
For example, as we discussed earlier, women in Marin County live at or below the federal poverty line at a rate of 15% more than men. Therefore, alleviating the factors that lead to people living in poverty (not just charitable support) inherently address gender inequality. And poverty is a factor contributing to SDGs #2, #3, and #4 as well. While housing is officially under SDG #11 Sustainable Cities and Communities (along with transportation and disaster preparedness), the Zillow study cited at the beginning of the chapter illustrates the obvious but often overlooked relationship between income, housing, and gender.

SDG #2 Zero Hunger and SDG #5 Gender Equality
While men, statistically speaking, are the greater "bread winners," nevertheless it is women who bear the greater responsibility for grocery shopping and food preparation. At the community level, food access issues are more of a problem for women and children than for men. Consider the following:

> *A systematic review assessing household food insecurity (primarily in the Americas and Europe) found that women were 40 percent more likely to report food insecurity, and that female-headed households were 75 percent more*

likely to be food insecure than male-headed households.
U.S. households with children have higher food insecurity
(13.9 percent) than those without (7.5 percent), and since
women are more likely to head single parent households,
they are at higher risk.[142]

Just as with poverty at large, food access and hunger are intimately tied to gender equality. The following is a quote that applies to present-day Marin County only in relatively small ways, given our modern lifestyle. However, considering the growing importance of local food production, and the fact that it illustrates the intimate connection between women and food production, I include it here for your consideration:

An FAO [Food and Agriculture Organization of the
United Nations] study suggests that if women had the
same access to productive resources as men, the production
of their farms would increase by 20-30%. This, in turn,
would increase agricultural production in developing
countries by 2.5-4% and decrease the number of hungry
people by 12%.[143]

---

142 Maryruth Belsey-Priebe, Deborah Lyons, and Jonathan J. Buonocore, "COVID-19's Impact on American Women's Food Insecurity Foreshadows Vulnerabilities to Climate Change," *International Journal of Environmental Research and Public Health* 18, no. 13 (June 26, 2021): 6867, https://doi.org/10.3390/ijerph18136867.

143 Carmen Rio and Lina Salazar, "What Is the Role of Women in Food Security," Inter-American Development Bank, October 2, 2017, https://blogs.iadb.org/sostenibilidad/en/cual-es-el-rol-de-la-mujer-en-la-seguridad-alimentaria-2/.

The article goes on to explain that ". . . it is poverty and not the availability of food that is the principal factor in food insecurity." This is true about Marin County as well: if you have money, you have ready access to nutritious food. The less money you have, the less access to quality food you have. Just as with poverty in general, social change that ensure that everyone has ready access to nutritious, quality food is a matter of gender equality.

SDG #3 Good Health & Well-Being and SDG #5 Gender Equality
As we saw in chapter three, African American women receive some of the lowest quality care in the healthcare environment, specifically with regard to prenatal outcomes. Earlier in this chapter, however, we noted that overall, women have slightly longer lifespans than men, both in Marin County and globally, indicating that there is a greater level of gender equality with regard to health. However, when it comes to people's lived experience within the healthcare system, women overall experience greater instances of gender discrimination than men:

One in five women say they have felt that a healthcare provider has ignored or dismissed their symptoms, and 17% say they feel they have been treated differently because of their gender—compared with 14% and 6% of men, respectively.[144]

---

144 Emily Paulsen, "Recognizing, Addressing Unintended Gender Bias in Patient Care," Duke Health Referring Physicians, January 14, 2020, https://physicians.dukehealth.org/articles/recognizing-addressing-unintended-gender-bias-patient-care.

SDG #5 GENDER EQUALITY

To clarify the quote above, 20% of women say they have experienced a healthcare provider ignoring or dismissing their symptoms, while 14% of men report similar experiences. Seventeen percent of women "say they have been treated differently because of their gender," while only 6% of men report the same.

Of course, we don't want *anyone* for any reason to experience what this quote describes: dismissal of their symptoms. As we covered in the SDG #3 chapter, our healthcare system is fraught with issues, and all in a context of *extremely* high cost. But as we see above, there is some evidence to indicate that this fraught system is even a bit more of a burden for women than for men. The article explains that there is a reason for the complaints of women in this case:

Studies show that women's perceptions of gender bias are correct. Compared with male patients, women who present with the same condition may not receive the same evidence-based care. In several key areas, such as cardiac care and pain management, women may get different treatment, leading to poorer outcomes.

Abortion rights also fall in this category of "cross-talk" between SDG #3 Good Health & Well-Being and #5 Gender Equality. Perhaps until we have equal pay, no more gender bias in the healthcare system, and gender-balanced domestic violence rates, men should step aside and let women decide whether or not abortion should be legal? In fact, perhaps only women who are or have been mothers should decide for the country if abortion should be legal? Mothers are, after all, the group with, collectively, the most insight into the process of conception, gestation, and birth, and the corresponding level of commitment required to supply a human child with a decent life.

SDG #4 Quality Education and SDG #5 Gender Equality
In the current and previous chapter, we have covered that quality education of women and girls through secondary school is a uniquely powerful point of influence when it comes to the quality of life for our whole society, with positive ecological outcomes as well. Delivering quality education to women and girls necessarily includes what is called "comprehensive sexuality education," a particularly rigorous form of family planning education, in addition to ready and reliable access to family planning services.

Interweaving Challenges & Solutions
In systems thinking we tend to avoid use of the term "solutions." A solution is usually thought of as a "fix" to a problem. In reality, however, the issues we are discussing in *Dear Marin* are all complex, and all involve living systems. We're not dealing with "problems" and "solutions" when it comes to poverty, food access, and overall human well-being. Rather, we're attempting to look at and understand what is going on, why, and how to improve circumstances for all in perpetuity.

How can Marin County meet Global Goal #5 Gender Equality? Ensure that every last woman and girl in Marin County has ready and reliable access to quality education, through secondary school. (Without solid basic education it is not impossible, but it is certainly more difficult, to continue education beyond high school.) Further, ensure she has access to quality, comprehensive family planning. But that doesn't just mean you need to provide schools and family planning centers. It means that our whole society is responsible for providing her and her family with the support systems they need—from nutritious food to reliable transportation and reasonable mental and physical healthcare and housing—to support her and her education. It means that we are all responsible for ensuring that she can walk into a family planning center that is easily accessible, and staffed with knowledgeable, culturally competent staff. We have decades of data to support the claim that when women and girls have these two things—quality education through secondary school and comprehensive family planning—the world changes *for everyone* for the better.

CHAPTER 6

SDG #6 Clean Water and Sanitation

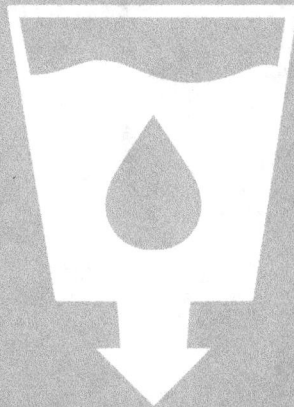

Where Are We?

The full text of this goal is, "Ensure availability and sustainable management of water and sanitation for all." Some of the targets of this Global Goal are aimed at providing a basic level of safe drinking water and reasonable sanitation for developing nations, but other targets have not been met even in places such as Marin County.

If you have lived or traveled in developing nations, particularly in poverty-stricken areas, then you are probably very grateful for the level of clean water and sanitation enjoyed by the Western world. The white, porcelain flushing toilet is one of the hallmarks of a "civilized" society. Similarly, the outhouse or a hole in the ground symbolizes poverty. And exactly how human waste is treated and stored influence whether or not you dare to drink water from the tap in your geographic location. . . if there *is* a tap. According to UNICEF, approximately 60% of the world (4.5 billion people) "don't have a toilet that safely manages human waste at home".[145] That's a lot of people.

"Open defecation" and other mismanagement (or no management) of human waste becomes a disease-spreading problem quite quickly. Again, according to UNICEF, more than 750 children younger than five-years-old die every single

---

145 "7 Fast Facts about Toilets," UNICEF, November 19, 2018, https://www.unicef.org/stories/7-fast-facts-about-toilets.

day due to "diarrhoea caused by unsafe water, sanitation, and poor hygiene."[146]

However, as we will see, even the developed West doesn't have water supply nor waste treatment, right. The visceral reaction we have to sewage has somehow served to undercut a truly sustainable way of handling and making the best use of our bodily wastes, and this in turn undermines what could be a far more sustainable water supply. We are missing out on opportunities to make the world a better place because of our huge, collective blind spot when it comes to feces and urine. Moreover, we are wasting resources in a waste management system that is ultimately profoundly wasteful itself, and inadequate. This is a major issue, particularly in the American Southwestern states that are in a perpetual drought.

In Marin, squandering resources is not, however, the only issue we have in this Global Goal area. Developed nations such as the United States are continuously adding contaminants to our freshwater systems, either on purpose (as "treatment") or as a byproduct of manufacturing or military activity. Even if we don't have military installations or large manufacturing in Marin County, we purchase food and consumer goods grown or manufactured irresponsibly, contributing to the degraded quality of our larger environment and other people's health. Nationwide, our waterways are used as a toilet for all kinds of dangerous substances. Historical and even current images of burning rivers reflect the continually challenging relationship we have to water.

---

146 Ibid.

"Clean Water and Sanitation," like all of the SDGs, is less a distinct category and more of a node that links multiple SDGs together. In particular, SDG #15 Life on Land comes into play, as this SDG deals with watersheds. There is an intimate, interconnected nature to both supplying clean water to communities and handling waste in a sanitary fashion. We will deal with these topics in this chapter both discreetly and together, as well as touching on stormwater and water pollution more generally.

Energy Use, Water, & Wastewater

According to the Environmental Protection Agency, wastewater and drinking water systems use around 2% of all energy consumed for any reason, resulting in 45 million tons of greenhouse gas emissions.[147] Two percent may seem small, but keep in mind we're talking about percentages here. This is the single largest source of energy use on the part of municipal governments, "accounting for 30 to 40 percent of total energy consumed."[148] That means that despite appearances, our drinking water and wastewater systems are massive consumers of electricity, which entails carbon output and ecological impact on a scale we can't really fathom. Whenever you turn on the faucet, the shower, flush the toilet or water the yard, you are contributing to carbon emissions, and global warming. If you are hooked up to alternative energy sources (and maybe even

---

147 "Energy Efficiency for Water Utilities," US EPA, March 30, 2022, https://www.epa.gov/sustainable-water-infrastructure/energy-efficiency-water-utilities.
148 Ibid.

a solar-powered well), as MCE here in Marin makes possible, your water use has less of a negative impact in terms of energy use. But we are still huge water wasters. This is less about household habits than it is about the system as a whole, including building codes and social norms.

Household Water Use

As consumers it can be tiresome being perpetually told to take five-minute showers and quit watering the lawn, especially when we hear about the outsized use of water by big agriculture and fracking. However, the fact remains that our present system of household water use is wasteful and down-right ridiculous.

Case in point: flushing our toilets with drinking water. Any glance at household water use data tells you immediately that the toilet is the largest consumer of water in your typical home. Personally, I think this echoes our anxiety about our "crap"; we have a clawing desire to "flush away" the icky stuff.

Another case in point: letting greywater go to waste. Our civilization has gone to great pains to get that bit of water to you, and then you hardly use it before you let it fall into the drain and out to the San Francisco Bay. In essence, we treat water as "disposable." The least you could do is use greywater to flush your toilet, and the majority of it should be watering your yard, helping to build soil and habitat, and grow food for you and local wildlife.

But is this situation your fault? Even if you are the one who built your home, is greywater even legal? It certainly isn't the norm. Recycled water system policy is set-aside, dealt with suspiciously as divergent from conventional plumbing and water system guidelines.

Later we will look at how to shift this from this wasteful use of water and energy to a more sustainable flow. It requires more than a shift in plumbing; it's a change in worldview.

Water Use & Sanitation in the United States: A Mixed Bag

WorldAtlas.com lists six rivers that have been known to catch on fire at least once. Of those, four are in the United States.[149] The most well-known is the Cuyahoga River in Cleveland, Ohio. Its first known fire was in 1868, and it burned 11 more times until 1969.[150] (Unfortunately, it caught on fire again August 25, 2020, when a tanker truck on the adjacent road spilled oil into it.) Water catching fire is only the most extreme manifestation of a legacy of abuse of our waterways in the United States: waterways that we depend on for all aspects of life.

The Water Research Foundation reports that per capita water use in the United States has been declining since the 1980s, due to improvements in efficiency and regulations, among other factors.[151] That's good news, because according

---

149 John Misachi, "Rivers That Have Caught On Fire," WorldAtlas, April 25, 2017, https://www.worldatlas.com/articles/is-the-cuyahoga-river-the-only-river-to-ever-catch-on-fire.html.

150 Wes Siler, "51 Years Later, the Cuyahoga River Burns Again," Outside Online, August 28, 2020, https://www.outsideonline.com/outdoor-adventure/environment/cuyahoga-river-fire-2020-1969/.

151 "Water Use and Efficiency," The Water Research Foundation, 2022, https://www.waterrf.org/sites/default/files/file/2022-03/4949-Water-Use-Efficiency.pdf.

to Water Footprint Calculator, only the United Arab Emirates uses more water per person per day (2,270 gallons) than the United States (2,200 gallons).[152] And we use about 24% more than the next most water use-intensive country, Canada (1,687 gallons).

The State of Water and Sanitation Infrastructure
According to a 2017 report from the Bipartisan Policy Center, water and sanitation infrastructure in the United States is in desperate need of upgrading. They describe the sheer scope of our national water and sanitation system:

> *. . . the United States has 1.2 million miles of water-supply mains—26 miles of water mains for every mile of interstate highway. That is just the drinking water system. There are nearly an equal number of sewer pipes.*
>
> *The nation has 14,478 POTWs [Publicly Owned Treatment Works] that serve more than 238 million Americans, or 76 percent of the U.S. population.*
>
> *There are approximately 52,000 CWSs [Community Water Systems] and 17,000 not-for-profit noncommunity water systems, including schools, and about 15 percent of the U.S. water market is privately owned.*[153]

---

152 "Water Footprint Comparisons by Country," Water Footprint Calculator, May 22, 2017, https://www.watercalculator.org/footprint/water-footprints-by-country/.

153 Steve Bartlet et al., *Understanding America's Water and Wastewater Challenges* (Washington, DC: Bipartisan Policy Center, 2017), 4.

The authors of the report explain the lack of coordination among the various entities responsible for sanitary, stormwater, and drinking water systems:

> *One might think wastewater, drinking water, and stormwater are all managed in a seamless system from water intake through the [Community Water System], into the home, out through the sewers into the [Publicly Owned Treatment Works], and back into the environment. . . in reality, very little coordination may exist among the entities that oversee the various parts of the process.*[154]

The report claims that people in the United States are accustomed to paying significantly less for water and wastewater services than in economically comparable nations, and that "Most rates paid by consumers today do not reflect the long-term costs of maintaining and repairing U.S. water and wastewater systems; often they are just a reflection of short-term construction and service cost."[155]

The authors paint a grim picture of the pollutants in the system, from the Flint Water crisis to drinking water violations across the nation and contaminated water making its way to human contact as a result of stormwater or other capacity issues:

---

154 Ibid., 9.
155 Ibid., 16.

The Environmental Protection Agency (EPA) estimates that between 1.8 million and 3.5 million people per year become ill from recreational contact, such as swimming, with water contaminated by overflows of sanitary sewers, which carry sewage to wastewater treatment plants. Furthermore, the American Society of Civil Engineers estimates that aging pipes and inadequate capacity result in the discharge of 900 billion gallons of untreated sewage into U.S. waterways each year.[156]

This document also cites estimates of loss of water from the systems due to old and failing infrastructure: "It has been estimated that the average system loses 16 percent of its water. . . "[157] For example, "The Chicago area alone loses 22 billion gallons of treated water per year through leaky pipes which could otherwise serve 698,000 people."[158]

Note that this outfit, the Bipartisan Policy Center, promotes the idea of the private sector getting more involved in water infrastructure. That means maximizing profit for shareholders in the private sector. Considering the systems thinking point about the "purpose" of a system covered earlier, this is a road that should be trod with extreme caution, if at all.

Native North Americans and Safe Drinking Water Access
In 2021 the *L.A. Times* reported that "58 out of every 1,000 Native American households don't have access to indoor

---

156 Ibid., 5.
157 Ibid., 17.
158 Ibid.

plumbing."[159] While Black and Latino households are twice as likely as White households to lack indoor plumbing, "Native American households are 19 times more likely than White households to lack indoor plumbing." They go on to cite the following:

About 130,150 out of 409,535 homes of Native Americans that the government organization Indian Health Service, or IHS, surveyed most recently needed sanitation facility improvements involving water, sewer or solid waste systems at the end of fiscal year 2018. The costs to improve these systems are an estimated $2.67 billion, according to the IHS.

According to the Public Policy Institute of California, there are 88 tribal water systems that together serve greater than 160,000 people. They cite a report from the State Water Board documenting 13 of those systems have contaminants that exceed state and federal drinking water standards, and another 22 are at risk of violations.[160]

---

159 Celina Tebor, "On Native American Reservations, the Push for More Clean Water and Sanitation," *Los Angeles Times*, June 26, 2021, sec. World & Nation, https://www.latimes.com/world-nation/story/2021-06-26/native-americans-clean-water.

160 "Ensuring Safe Drinking Water for California's Native American Communities," Public Policy Institute of California, June 22, 2021, https://www.ppic.org/blog/ensuring-safe-drinking-water-for-californias-native-american-communities/.

Water Use in California

> *We have forgotten that the natural West is bar-*
> *ren, and fatally dry, and that our new, bountiful*
> *West is a fragile construction.*[161]
>
>   —Cadillac Desert

In 2018 the California state legislature passed a bill that in theory limits per capita indoor water use to 55 gallons per person per day. There is no method or budget for monitoring or enforcing that basic idea included in the bill, so it remains largely a guideline for utilities (we don't currently have a way of separating out indoor versus outdoor water use). In 2022 the guideline was lowered in the state Senate to 47 gallons, and of this writing it is unknown whether this update will pass the Assembly.

Despite the largely representative nature of this bill, it nevertheless illustrates that California is a very dry state, and officials are concerned. When urban water use rose in March of 2022, up by 19% compared with March of 2020,[162] alarm bells went off. In May of 2022, the Metropolitan Water District of Southern California started publicly discussing

---

161 Jkoomjian, "Cadillac Desert - 1. Mulhollands Dream (1 of 9)," YouTube, April 10, 2010, https://www.youtube.com/watch?v=hkbebOhnCjA.

162 Rachel Ramirez, "California Is in a Water Crisis, yet Usage Is Way up. Officials Are Focusing on the Wrong Things, Advocates Say - CNN," CNN, May 15, 2022, https://edition.cnn.com/2022/05/15/us/california-water-usage-increase-drought-climate/index.html.

unprecedented water regulations, such as the possibility of a complete ban on outdoor watering by September 1st.[163]

The classic book and film *Cadillac Desert: The American West and It's Disappearing Water,* is a long-standing reference for understanding the century-long efforts to bring water to the dry West. In part it documents the vision of explorer John Wesley Powell, who in 1888 warned the U.S. Congress about the profound lack of water in the Southwest. Powell created a fascinating, unprecedented map of the Western states with the colored area indicating regional watersheds. It was the first-ever map of its kind. It is described in a book about Powell:

> *Here he displayed a map of the arid lands, separated into colorful circles of various sizes, designating watersheds. He also introduced the idea of irrigation districts, which would manage their own water, neither sending it out of their own watershed nor importing any from another.*[164]

---

163 Stephanie Elam, "Officials Worry Southern California Won't Have Enough Water to Get Through Summer Without Unprecedented Cuts," CNN, May 4, 2022, https://www.cnn.com/2022/05/04/us/california-drought-water-restrictions-climate/index.html.

164 John F. Ross, *The Promise of the Grand Canyon: John Wesley Powell's Perilous Journey and His Vision for the American West* (New York, New York: Viking, 2018), 308.

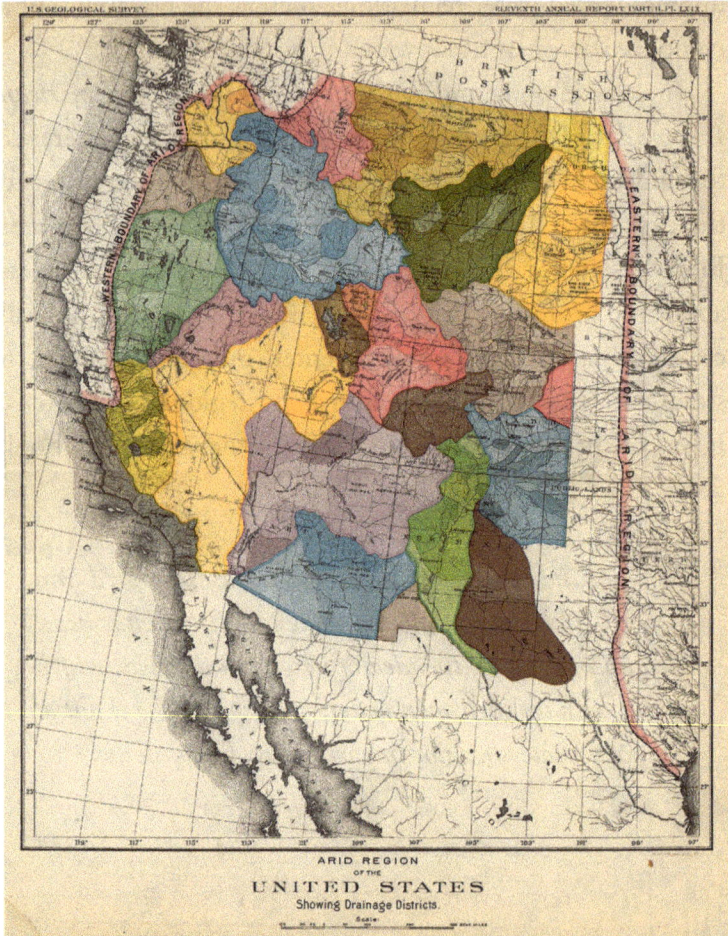

Figure 17 - Torpyl, CC BY-SA 4.0, via Wikimedia Commons

Unfortunately, Congress ignored Powell's recommendations, overriding nature with massive waterworks on a scale never before seen in human history, bringing us to the situation documented in *Cadillac Desert*.

Cadillac Desert: A Case Study in Systems Thinking
Water and water supply is a helpful example when trying to
understand what "systems thinking" really is. Referencing
Systems Thinking: A Primer, *Cadillac Desert* provides ample
examples of what Donella Meadows describes as "systems traps."

Of the eight systems traps, *Cadillac Desert* includes at least
four of them, and arguably more. I'll leave it to you to discover
the plethora of examples in the film (or the book), but here is
one example.

The government-funded waterworks documented in
Cadillac Desert enabled millions of new people to settle in
new lands over a hundred years. These lands don't have reliable, naturally occurring water supplies to support millions of
people (or that much agriculture) within hundreds of miles.
The projects, one after the other over the decades, made this
possible.

Each time a new project went into effect, it alleviated the
current need for water, yet engendered space for more water
need in the form of more agricultural activity, and more people.

This cycle has been repeating itself over and over again since
the early 1900s.

There is a simple word for this: addiction. But there is also
a more specific systems trap label: "Shifting the Burden to the
Intervenor."

Shifting the Burden to the Intervenor
The name of this systems trap encapsulates the *Cadillac Desert*
scenario. The only entity robust enough to intervene on the
scale necessary to bring water to the dry Southwest was the

United States government. Sufficiently poked and prodded by special interests, paired with some sincere care and desire to help people, dreams were realized.

But the dreams quickly turned nightmarish. And rather than stepping back and finding a different way, perhaps more commensurate with Powell's recommendations, the same mistake has been repeated over and over for decades, right up to the present day.

Meadows defines Shifting the Burden to the Intervenor:

A well-meaning and efficient intervenor watches the struggle and steps in to take some of the load. The intervenor quickly brings the system to the state everybody wants it to be in. Congratulations are in order...

Then the original problem reappears, since nothing has been done to solve it at its root cause. So the intervenor applies more of the "solution," disguising the real state of the system again, and thereby failing to act on the problem. That makes it necessary to use still more "solution."[165]

The description so far describes a cyclical process, a downward spiral that one can imagine in any addiction process. The "trap" aspect actually comes in later.

The trap is formed if the intervention, whether by active destruction or simple neglect, undermines the original

---

165 Donella Meadows, *Thinking in Systems: International Bestseller* (New York: Chelsea Green Publishing, 2008), 135.

capacity of the system to maintain itself. If that capacity atrophies, then more of the intervention is needed to achieve the desired effect.[166]

She asks, "Why does anyone enter the trap?" Whether motivated by profit-seeking, or genuine goodwill toward a group in need, a lack of foresight and a lack of a systems view is the problem.

Meadows explains what should happen instead:

The problem can be avoided up front by intervening in such a way as to strengthen the ability of the system to shoulder its own burdens. This option, helping the system to help itself, can be much cheaper and easier than taking over and running the system—something liberal politicians don't seem to understand.[167]

Her little jab there at the end could indeed be applied across the aisle; often the reasons for allocating funds are cloaked in arguments for "jobs." In this case, the system 'shouldering its own burdens' would be human settlements adjusting their water needs to meet the relatively local supply. Our country as a whole, however, is the very embodiment of precisely the opposite of this principle: globalizing supply chains to the degree that formerly local supply chains (or ecosystem services) are neglected, overrun, or obsolete, and often breakdown

---

166 Ibid.
167 Ibid., 154.

altogether. The warnings of people like Powell were left in the dust. Certain areas of California and the West are simply running out of water.[168]

Running Out of Water
More water could be found and piped in from even further away. Doing so would be the embodiment of the same mindset that led to the present-day conundrums in the first place: a linear view demanding a bandage approach that further exacerbates the problem, laying the groundwork for catastrophe on an even greater scale in the future.

The image below, from the California State Department of Water Resources, illustrates that between 2001 and 2021 the overall trend of groundwater levels in California is that they are sinking (sometimes causing "subsidence," that is, the land sinking down due to the disappearance of the water under them). The report authors state, ". . . water levels in more than 55 percent of statewide wells demonstrate a decreasing trend and just over six percent of wells demonstrate an increasing trend."[169]

168 Rachel Ramirez, "As California's Big Cities Fail to Rein in Their Water Use, Rural Communities Are Already Tapped Out," CNN, June 6, 2022, https://edition.cnn.com/2022/06/05/us/california-rural-groundwater-crisis-climate/index.html

169 Gavin Newsom, "Groundwater Conditions Report Water Year 2021" (California Natural Resources Agency, 2021), 11, https://water.ca.gov/-/media/DWR-Website/Web-Pages/Programs/Groundwater-Management/Data-and-Tools/Files/Statewide-Reports/Groundwater-Conditions-Report-Fall-2021.pdf.

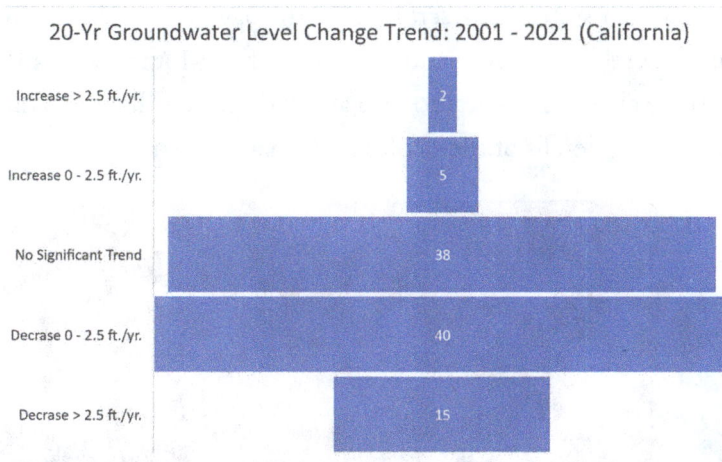

Figure 18 - Data from the California State Department of Water Resources, 2001 - 2021

Urban areas are less vulnerable to groundwater levels due to the dependence on large waterworks importing water. It is families, small farmers and wildlife and the environment who depend on local water. Even today new wells are being installed in California, further exacerbating water loss.

Clean Water & Sanitation in Marin County

Drought

If you're ever wondering whether or not your area is technically considered in a drought or not at any given time, you can go to this website to investigate. The National Integrated Drought Information System at drought.gov allows you to look up your state, city, or zip code. Click on "By Location" in the menu and select your state. Then, scroll down the page to reveal a handy map like the one below, and click on your area for more details. (These charts are easiest to read at a glance: we will discuss the confusing details of their color scale in a moment.)

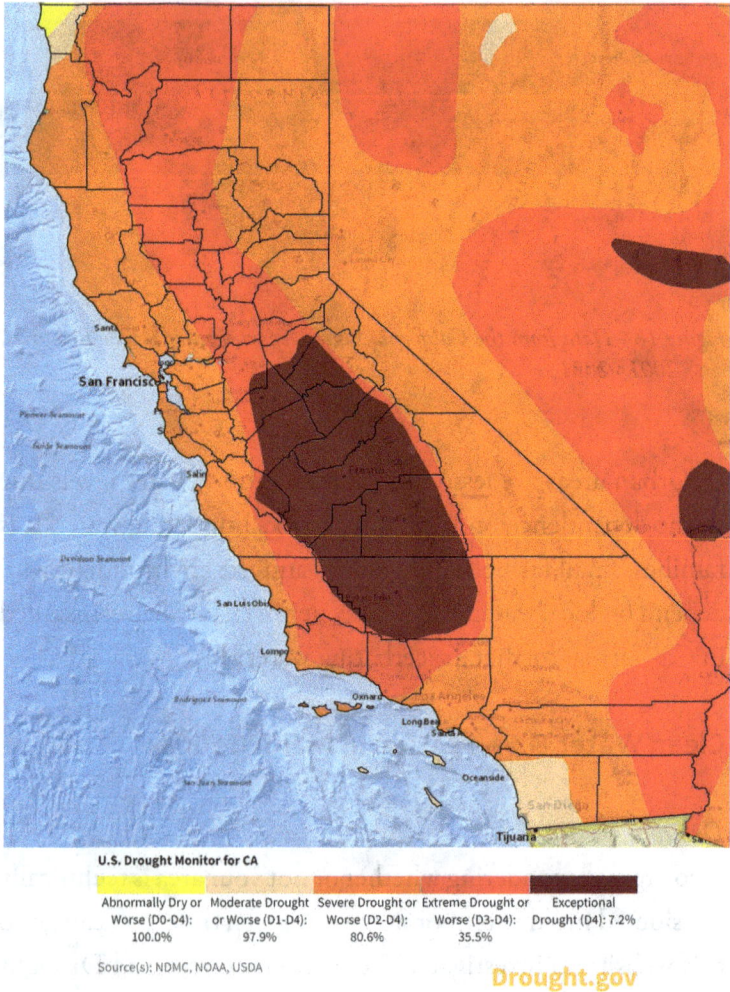

U.S. Drought Monitor for CA

Abnormally Dry or Worse (D0-D4): 100.0%	Moderate Drought or Worse (D1-D4): 97.9%	Severe Drought or Worse (D2-D4): 80.6%	Extreme Drought or Worse (D3-D4): 35.5%	Exceptional Drought (D4): 7.2%

Source(s): NDMC, NOAA, USDA

Drought.gov

Figure 19 - National Integrated Drought Information System, California, August 2022

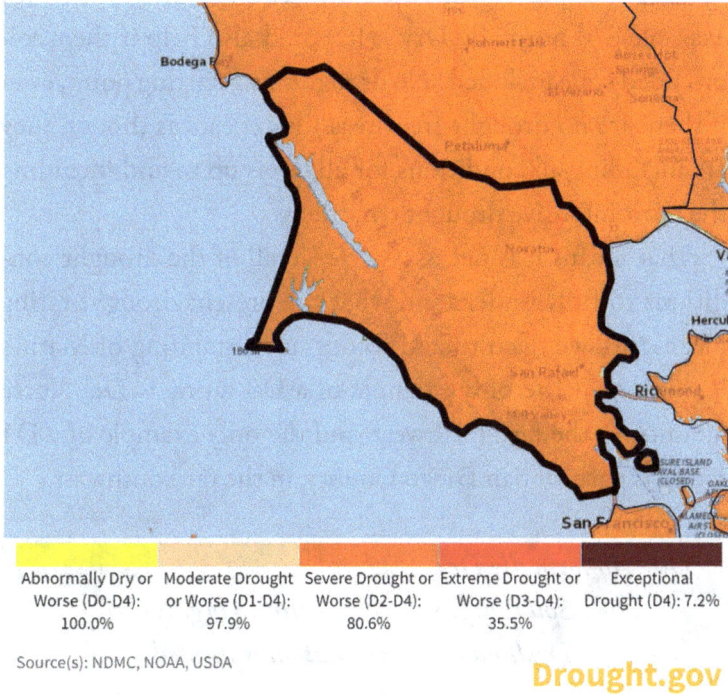

| Abnormally Dry or Worse (D0-D4): 100.0% | Moderate Drought or Worse (D1-D4): 97.9% | Severe Drought or Worse (D2-D4): 80.6% | Extreme Drought or Worse (D3-D4): 35.5% | Exceptional Drought (D4): 7.2% |

Source(s): NDMC, NOAA, USDA

Drought.gov

Figure 20 - National Integrated Drought Information System, Marin County, August 2022

As they say, a picture is worth a thousand words. According to this website, Marin County is in a "D2" or "Severe" drought as of this writing (Autumn 2022). The conditions listed for severe drought are the following:

- *Grazing land is inadequate*
- *Fire season is longer, with high burn intensity, dry fuels, and large fire spatial extent*
- *Trees are stressed, wildlife diseases increase*

I for one was confused by the "100%" figure under, for example, "Abnormally Dry." (It would also help if their color-coded scale included "No drought" as a starting point, even if there are no drought-free areas.) It appears as though they are including all conditions for all levels up to and including the most intensive drought condition.

That means it is necessary to read all of the drought conditions to fully understand what the present drought rating means. So, we need to add to our understanding of Marin's conditions. (The only example of a D0 rating is Del Norte County, in the far Northwest, and the only example of a D1 rating is parts of San Diego County, in the far Southwest.)

D0 - Abnormally Dry
- *Soil is dry; irrigation delivery begins early*
- *Dryland crop germination is stunted*
- *Active fire season begins*

D1 - Moderate Drought
- *Dryland pasture growth is stunted; producers give supplemental feed to cattle*
- *Landscaping and gardens need irrigation earlier; wildlife patterns begin to change*
- *Stock ponds and creeks are lower than usual*

If that isn't depressing enough, for comparison you can look at counties such as Mariposa, 100% of which is in Extreme Drought, and 90.23% of which is listed in "Exceptional Drought."

D3 - Extreme Drought

- *Livestock need expensive supplemental feed; cattle and horses are sold; little pasture remains; fruit trees bud early; producers begin irrigating in the winter*
- *Fire season lasts year-round; fires occur in typically wet parts of state; burn bans are implemented*
- *Water is inadequate for agriculture, wildlife, and urban needs; reservoirs are extremely low; hydropower is restricted*

D4 - Exceptional Drought

- *Fields are left fallow; orchards are removed; vegetable yields are low; honey harvest is small*
- *Fire season is very costly; number of fires and area burned are extensive*
- *Fish rescue and relocation begins; pine beetle infestation occurs; forest mortality is high; wetlands dry up; survival of native plants and animals is low; fewer wildflowers bloom; wildlife death is widespread; algae blooms appear*

This database provides a variety of additional data and graphics. One of the graphics is the "Historical Conditions" graph.

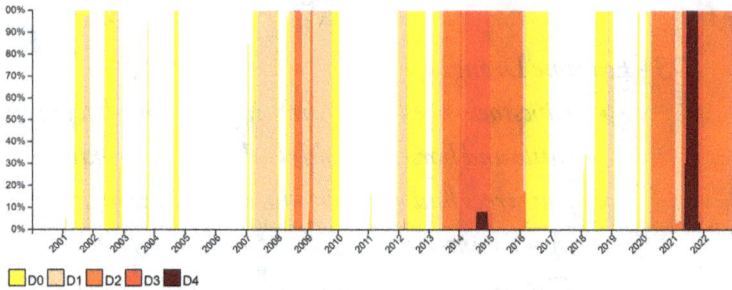

Figure 21 - National Integrated Drought Information System, Marin County, 2001 to 2022

This data shows a general trend, on a weekly basis, toward more frequent and more intense droughts between the years of 2000 and 2022. We can see this based on the greater prevalence of darker vertical bars towards the right side, or the more recent end of the chart.

Contamination

Of course, we want to be responsibly managing the water that we *do* have, especially in areas of drought. In the San Geronimo Creek, here in the San Geronimo Valley, studies have found bacteria from human waste in the waters of the creek.[170] The June 29th edition of the *Pacific Sun* featured a cover story titled, "Don't Drink the Water: Marin City's Contaminated Water and the District's Denials." The tiny water districts of Nicasio Valley Ranch Mutual and the Nicasio School have known water quality violations, as reported on the California

---

170 "The Woodacre/San Geronimo Flats Wastewater Group," Woodacre/San Geronimo Flats Wastewater Group, September 2018, http://www. woodacresangeronimoflats.org/links/_pdf/Sept2018-Newsletter.pdf.

Water Board's website.[171] And the Environmental Working Group (EWG) "Tap Water Database" lists 24 contaminants found in Marin Municipal Water District's (MMWD) water, 12 of which exceed guidelines set by EWG.[172] For comparison purposes, Petaluma's Tap Water Database results include 29 total contaminants with 13 exceeding EWG guidelines,[173] San Francisco has 13 total contaminants with five exceeding guidelines,[174] and East Bay Municipal Utility District has 14 total with three exceeding EWG guidelines.[175]

I spoke with a friend whose water was tested as part of the Marin City water quality investigation as reported in the *Pacific Sun* article. Happily, my friend's tap water test results came out negative for any of the elements in question. However, together we also looked at the EWG database for MMWD water. EWG explains graphically that "Legal ≠ Safe."

EWG Health Guidelines fill the gap in outdated government standards. The federal government's legal limits are

171 "Information for Public Drinking Water Systems," California State Water Resources Control Board, accessed August 28, 2022, https://www.waterboards.ca.gov/drinking_water/certlic/drinkingwater/2022.html.

172 "Marin Municipal Water District."

173 "City of Petaluma," Environmental Working Group, accessed August 28, 2022, https://www.ewg.org/tapwater/system.php?pws=CA4910006?pws=CA4910006.

174 "San Francisco City Water System," Environmental Working Group, accessed August 28, 2022, https://www.ewg.org/tapwater/system.php?pws=CA3810011?pws=CA3810011.

175 "East Bay Municipal Utility District," Environmental Working Group, accessed August 28, 2022, https://www.ewg.org/tapwater/system.php?pws=CA0110005?pws=CA0110005.

DEAR MARIN

not health-protective. The EPA has not set a new tap water standard in almost 20 years, and some standards are more than 40 years old.[176]

Bromochloroacetic acid

Just to take one example, EWG lists bromochloroacetic acid found in the MMWD water supply at 200x the EWG recommendation. Bromochloroacetic acid is an example not of a pollutant found naturally, nor as a result of human activity that inadvertently pollutes bodies of water, but rather, is created during water treatment.

> *Bromochloroacetic acid is formed when chlorine or other disinfectants are used to treat drinking water. Bromochloroacetic acid and other disinfection byproducts increase the risk of cancer and may cause problems during pregnancy.*[177]

That is, our utility isn't intentionally adding Bromochloroacetic acid into the water supply, but rather, the chemicals they *do* intentionally add in order to disinfect our water supply lead to the presence of this byproduct.

Bromochloroacetic acid is listed as a "Group 2B carcinogen." This grouping schema is a classification provided by the International Agency for Research on Cancer of the World Health Organization. Group 2B is considered "possibly

---

176 "Marin Municipal Water District."
177 Ibid.

carcinogenic to humans" as distinguished from Group 2A which is defined as "probably carcinogenic to humans."[178]

EWG has detected bromochloroacetic acid in 24 states, and 4,566 water utilities (serving 55 million people), most of which are in Texas (2,474), and a smaller number in California (192), in addition to a handful of other states. EWG recommends a limit of 0.02 parts per billion (ppb). MMWDs water supply test results show 3.99 ppb. For comparison purposes, the highest single instance reported in the EWG database is the Snyder Public Works Authority in Snyder, Oklahoma, at 27.7 ppb.[179]

Of course, this isn't a concern just for Marin City's water supply, but for all of the MMWD service area.

Our Local Water Districts
Nevertheless, in many ways we are fortunate here in Marin County with regard to water resources. MMWD, which supplies water for central and southern Marin, stewards a water district with seven reservoirs on 22,000 acres. The water itself is 75% the result of local rainfall.[180] Supplementary water to the districts comes from the Russian River. MMWD provides

178 World Health Organization, "IARC Monographs on the Evaluation of Carcinogenic Risks to Humans" (Lyon, France: World Health Organization, 2006).

179 "Bromochloroacetic Acid," Environmental Working Group, accessed August 28, 2022, https://www.ewg.org/tapwater/contaminant. php?contamcode=2455?contamcode=2455.

180 "2021 - Annual Water Quality Report," Marin Water, 2021, https:// www.marinwater.org/sites/default/files/2022-04/Esp%20-%20 AWQR%2004.28.22%20Web%20Ready.pdf.

a printed and online annual Water Quality Report, in both English and Spanish, with detailed data on the amounts of regulated contaminants found in our local water supply, and five un-regulated contaminants. Not only do we get relatively decent quality drinking water, but we also get the benefits of acres and acres of open space and recreational areas provided by the necessity of managing our pleasant lakes and surrounding lands.

The North Marin Water District (NMWD) provides the City of Novato and most of West Marin with water. The majority of this water is sourced from outside of the county.

Finally, there are some small, independent water district areas for Muir, Stinson, and Dillon Beach, as well as Bolinas. They rely on local groundwater.

Where do we want to get to?

As with all of the SDGs, the targets under this Goal are a great starting place for describing where we want to get to in this area, both nationally and locally. To paraphrase the targets under SDG #6, we want everyone to have ready access to clean water and sanitation, especially the most vulnerable; we want to drastically reduce the pollution from all sources currently contaminating our limited water supply and vastly increase water recycling; we have to protect and restore freshwater supplies, including groundwater, and the ecosystems that depend on these watersheds, and we need whole communities to be actively involved if we are going to make these positive changes.

But a deep worldview shift is in order for these targets to be met, much less exceeded. Water is currently commoditized. That may not be a sustainable schema. Water should be seen as something bordering on sacred, if not flat-out a gift from the gods. Anything short of a semi-sacred view of water simply may not be enough to sufficiently alter our collective relationship to it.

A sacred view of water is not a stretch. In fact, I would argue that most people already hold some notion of water as sacred, but that their instinct to revere and appreciate water is eroded by modern civilization and the enclosed, nearly invisible state of our current waterworks system.

So where do we want to get to? We want to unlock the power of our own sense of the sacred view of water that we already hold, and thereby have a much stronger chance of meeting the water targets. With this larger sense of transcendent meaning opened up, those targets under this SDG have a very different flavor. They seem to come alive as obvious. Of *course* everyone should have access to clean freshwater. Of *course* we don't want to pollute the waters we have. This becomes self-evident when we allow ourselves to enter into a different worldview; one that steps outside of the strictly logical mind and into a much larger experience of life, and water as a *whole* system.

How do we get there?

In a word: feedback loops. Donella Meadows discusses the crucial role of feedback loops in *Thinking In Systems: A Primer.* If we look at the water systems within which we exist right now, despite the incredible centrality of water to our lives and work, there are scant feedback loops in place to ensure that the average citizen is in the know about their water supply, or quality.

I live in the San Geronimo Valley. Short of knowing that the Marin Municipal Water District exists, and that there are some local lakes, I couldn't tell you off the top of my head precisely where my water comes from. And I'm someone who cares, a lot.

Rather than the latest shenanigans of national politicians or some vapid celebrity, the front page of our virtual and physical news sources should be a veritable dashboard of things like the state of our water supply (not just when there is a dramatic problem afoot). This version of reality would require a big shift in the "purpose" of our chosen media sources. The shift would be from news media sources that, due to their profit-as-the-priority business model (which is almost all news media) to media sources that—through their organizational structure—have enshrined community well-being as the top priority. Rather than a deluge of clickbait we engage with addictively and reflexively call "news," our news experience might be something more like that of an active participant in the world who is checking in on the state of local events so as to adjust and respond accordingly.

Imagine your day does not start with national or international news, but instead, with local news. Imagine that the current state of local water reservoirs is a factoid you conscientiously attend to as normal part of your week.

If we bump up our sense of the sacred and reverence for water, then almost miraculously, our sense of the *system* comes to the fore. Why? Simply because our "care" muscles get involved. Consider this quote from Obi Kaufman's lovely little book, *The State of Water: Understanding California's Most Precious Resource:*

> *Reservoirs behind hydroelectric dams expel large amounts of methane gas, a key climate-change contributor. To make matters worse, toxic algae from reservoirs is a problem for wildlife habitat and our health, and bacteria present in decaying vegetation can make mercury in the bedrock under a reservoir water-soluble.*[181]

If we look at this from a conventional, or what I would call a "linear" perspective, it's rather complicated and confounding. Even hydroelectric power has its problems, and significant problems at that. We quickly start to have a conversation about whether these drawbacks are worth the cost due to the urgency of climate change, i.e., how *much* methane and how *much* mercury are we talking about?

But if we back up and try on this much larger systems perspective, and a sense of reverence for, as Obi calls it, "California's most precious resource," then something else emerges. There's something about large hydroelectric dams that just doesn't *feel* right, such that the drawbacks that he is pointing to somehow seem less surprising. *Small* hydroelectric seems more... appropriate. Taking out dams and allowing the

---

181 Obi Kaufmann, *The State of Water: Understanding California's Most Precious Resource* (London: Heyday, 2019), 58.

fish to run *feels* a lot better. Reckoning with local water limits and finding ways to live within limits speaks to our inherent sense of responsibility.

In short, allowing in a sense of the sacred, and the depth of care that comes with it, expands my field of vision. And this vision is another version of intelligence; a higher, more sophisticated intelligence, paired with simple concern for the well-being of others.

If I *care* about water, I am curious about the state of our local reservoir after the last rainstorm. If I *care* about local wildlife, I would like to see in a glance if the fish have started back into my local creek yet, and if not, if there is anything I can do to help.

In this schema I am laying out, with a sense of the sacred paired with a knowledge of local systems, I get to be curious about my local ecology and social body, and have that curiosity satisfied. I have readily available data at hand, provided by intact and appropriately functioning feedback loops that are a product of a responsible civilization monitoring its own life support system on a continual basis.

Conclusion

This book deals with complex systems; that is, systems of living beings. As such, there are no easy answers and no ultimate solutions for any of these topics. Due to the nature of life ongoing, our concern is not "solutions" but rather, "evolution."

If evolving toward greater well-being is our *purpose*, then the Global Goals make good sense. If our purpose is profit and growth, then they really don't. These are two very different purposes, and as such, are incompatible.

Again, that doesn't mean you can't make money *and* help the planet and society to some limited extent. Rather, it means that if you sincerely want to help make the world a better place, you have to make *that* your purpose, clearly and unequivocally.

Infinite economic growth in the context of finite systems (that are interruptible and even breakable) is a fantasy of an extremely limited mental construct, a worldview with no real relationship to life. It touts slogans like, "It's easy being green!" and pawns products like "clean coal." It gives rise to a food system that adds to poverty, obesity and disease. A "health-care" system that is really "sick care." An educational system that is stuck in the industrial or even pre-industrial age, dragging down our economy, not to mention our youth. It gives rise to gender norms that are improving, and yet, somehow perennially backward. It's a worldview that pumps freshwater to neighborhoods and then back out again before it's hardly been used yet is now contaminated with feces. It lets water and energy-intensive food products become pollutants rather than converting the human manure into soil amendments for the local land. And then it sells you chemical fertilizers for your landscaping.

Out of this mindset also comes topics we don't deal with directly in this book; they are the purview of later SDGs. For example, if you look at #16 Peace, Justice, and Strong Institutions, you may find yourself asking, "What is the *purpose* of the police force?" As we have reviewed, to answer that question, you would not refer to slogans, but rather, you would look at what that system is actually producing. (Incidentally, you may check out a Radiolab episode that originally aired October 20, 2020, titled "No Special Purpose," about the police.[182])

Systems Take Aways
While *Dear Marin* is heavy on data points, what I really hope you take away are the systems thinking pointers. These are the aspects that will enable you to look at a current situation and see what you haven't noticed previously. They help to make the invisible more tangible; to see the unexpected connections between seemingly unrelated aspects, and to more intelligently attempt to aim toward—as Capra and Luisi say—"disturb" the

---

182 Radiolab, "No Special Duty," Radiolab, October 2, 2020, https://www.radiolab.org/episodes/no-special-duty.

system, rather than trying to force it to fit your view of what it "should" look like.[183]

Returning to Meadows' *Thinking in Systems,* systems thinking asks us to move into the realm of the unknown and to actively embrace uncertainty. I can't stress enough how contrary to business-as-usual this is. Most of us—individually and collectively—are fixated on control in some form or fashion. Embracing uncertainty is not about "throwing caution to the wind" wholesale. Rather, we follow through; we bring our best selves to our work. But we *nearly* anticipate that things will, in fact, "go wrong," and when they do, we let curiosity and humility get the better of us.

Sometimes we fixate on control and certainty not because we personally are committed to control and certainty, but because we feel the pressure of expectations and obligations on our shoulders, and *that* leads us to behave in ways we really don't believe in. Our institutions are built on a worldview that calls for and relies on maximizing certainty. This is a trap; it's a trap that has led us to the socially and ecologically unsustainable situation we find ourselves in today, such that we look at the Sustainable Development Goals and think they are quaint, though not particularly realistic. We think, "Well, that would be nice, to end poverty." But we really don't embrace that vision, the message, the possibility.

Embrace the possibility. Step into uncertainty. Wield your care for Marin, and for the world.

---

183 Fritjof Capra and Pier Luigi Luisi, *The Systems View of Life: A Unifying Vision* (Cambridge: Cambridge University Press, 2014), 256.

Epilogue

While I wrote this book for Marin County residents, for the benefit of the land and the people, the larger society and world were never far from my mind. Again, while Marin County is legitimately special in many ways, for the most part we are part and parcel of our larger human system, and our social and ecological outcomes are very much aligned with those of our country, and the world. The exceptions to this are extremely few and relatively minor.

I'm finishing up the edits to, and publication of *Dear Marin* in Pittsburgh, Pennsylvania. Driving across the country to arrive here was a feast of social and ecological vignettes that kept me reflecting on the Sustainable Development Goals as we went. We experienced the stark, arid beauty of the Western states. . . after we escaped the wildfire smoke that plagued us nearly all of the way through the state of Nevada. Colorado welcomed us with glorious colors and rainbows, but if we considered altering our ultimate destination, tales of a wildfire the week before—and a glance at real estate prices—kept us on track. Salt Lake City, Utah and Omaha, Nebraska were lovely cities that supplied us with trendy vegan restaurants and vistas of lightning. Saint Louis, Missouri kicked us out before we could hardly land—due to extreme air freshener in our accommodations and concern about the likelihood our car would make it through the night if left on the street in this run-down, sketchy neighborhood—but a little town outside of the city was welcoming and pleasant. A seemingly ancient tavern in Yellow Springs, Ohio was like being back in Europe, made even more colorful by a young gentleman who "just got out of jail" relaying his life story to a cop on the sidewalk. Bloomington, Indiana features a growing homeless population, something residents tell me is very new.

Having arrived in Pittsburgh mere weeks ago, we have already experienced some minor and major hiccups related to social and ecological issues in this city. It's a lovely, moderately-sized city with a lot to write home about. The people who live here have a lot of nice things to say about it. But our second morning in our new apartment was beset with the pervasive smell of hydrogen sulfide throughout the neighborhood, a result of winds blowing in the effluent from the still-functioning steel mill three miles from our house. (Why didn't anyone tell us before we signed a lease?) Nearly every night and morning since features the smell, though it often dissipates by late morning. We are advised by our landlords to use the air conditioning in the winter when the radiators get to be too much, which strikes me as an absurd imbroglio of inefficient infrastructure lacking basic feedback loops. But when you wake up at 2:30 AM and your bedroom is 75-degrees Fahrenheit (though it may be 20-degrees outside) and your Purple Air map is deep orange, on the AC goes.

These and more challenges I am not too surprised by. Our society's use of resources mimics the value we put on people: profit-driven, inefficient, outdated, lacking in basic creativity and care. Yet, to reference Theory U again, we are collectively creating outcomes that no one wants. Yes, a relatively small handful of people benefit from business as usual, but even their interests are ultimately undermined by an unsustainable world. So we are faced with a strange situation: our ongoing participation in a set of systems that, *en mass*, most people generally don't agree with.

The "solution" here is to clarify. Whether in Pittsburgh, Pennsylvania or Marin County, California, are we going to keep telling ourselves that we care about the environment and people while continuing to use so-called "natural gas" and voting against affordable housing? Are we going to continue thinking of ourselves as "progressive" while sitting back and allowing the expansion of roads over the improvement of public transport? Are we going to continue perpetuating gender inequity through subtle (or not so subtle) favoring of males over females in the workplace and our households? Are we going to keep berating our kids for failing to flourish in a backward (oh-so-backward) educational system, rather than advocating for high quality project-based learning in the school systems?

These things and more require abject, nearly cruel levels of clarity and self-reflection. Sometimes honesty, especially with yourself, can hurt. But just as we need to cultivate active and out-loud compassion for others, so too we need to hold our little selves with thoughtfulness even as we administer the medicine of clear thinking.

Acknowledgements

I primarily want to acknowledge the thousands of Marin County residents (and people who are otherwise invested in Marin as part of the large community) who, over the decades, have participated in workshop after workshop (after workshop) and survey after survey (after survey) and feel like your input didn't really make a difference; that the county is still as it's always been, or worse. Little trickles of your input appear in this book in the form of "data" cited from NGO or government agency reports. I hope that we collectively find ways to prioritize human and ecological well-being over profit and growth so that your voices become elevated as primary.

And I want to acknowledge to people in charge of those efforts who meant well and thought they were helping, many of whom became frustrated and changed careers, some of whom are still trying.

Special thank you to UNA Marin, especially Bonnie!

Many thanks to Tricia, Cornelius, Don McCray, Sunny, to Pam and the team at Inquiring Systems Inc., to that sharp scallywag Ricardo and fearless, delightful Elberta, to my reliable supporter Maralisia for your provocative input, and to Kyle and Anna for much needed, last-minute professional help. Thanks to the County of Marin's "Community Service Fund" for $3,000 toward this book project. And thank you to Stacey for your support with SDGMarin.org and early draft input.

And finally, to the trees, the beings, the waters, and the skies of Marin and beyond. As someone who primarily identifies as an environmentalist, you are my ultimate measure of worth, wellness, and joy.

Appendix A

Note: As a participant in Elberta Eriksson's Southern Marin Multi-Disciplinary Team meeting for two years, I repeatedly heard complaints from social service providers about barriers to their ability to serve their clients. This led to me working directly with a local provider who had experience in the past working in county social services. We drafted a statement to reflect her experience and the experiences I had heard from others, with the idea it would be reviewed, edited, and signed by a collective. (She in particular provided the bullet points to this statement.) It did not go beyond the MDT group, but I provide it here for your reference.

"As social service providers in Marin County we are prevented from optimally serving our clients by system constraints that do more harm than good."

As social service providers in Marin County, we are making this public statement in the interest of bringing greater awareness to a stark reality, and to spur movement toward positive change. As individuals we hope to make a positive difference in the world by entering this line of work. As service providers in Marin County, we are prevented from optimally serving our clients by system constraints that do more harm than good. We see the potential for improvements on a regular basis, but as practitioners we largely lack the leverage to implement changes. These conditions lead to service providers suffering from burnout, funding spent unwisely, and individuals and families lose out. Both practitioners and those we serve deserve better. While these conditions are not unique to Marin and obstacles beyond our local system are significant, we see the potential to collectively build a better, genuinely supportive social services system right here in this county.

The following is a list of examples of system constraints that negatively impact practitioners and clients:

- The mental health model followed by most county funded agencies is a medical model. This model requires clinicians to diagnose without enough knowledge of the client, often on the 1st or 2nd session. A mental health misdiagnoses can be extremely disempowering and have a life-long negative impact on the client's life and recovery process.
- The moral/ethical values of clinicians and other service providers, and the agencies/organizations for who they work for are mis-aligned. The medical model in mental health requires clinicians to focus most of their working hours doing documentation for funding and/or insurance requirements, rather than connecting with the client to understand and serve their needs.
- Mental health clinicians and service providers represent and/or are often seen as part of a system that has historically been abusive and oppressive towards underserved and underprivileged communities.

- Treatment models used across most county funded mental health agencies do not acknowledge the impact of systemic abuse and other forms of trauma in mental health.
- There is a lack of psychoeducation in treatment plan models. Psychoeducation about symptoms and their relationship to trauma, empowers clients to be in control of their healing process.

APPENDIX B

Note: From 2018 to 2022 I worked directly with and supported Ricardo Moncrief's ISOJI group; a community organization with a monthly public meeting in Marin City (during the pandemic, on Zoom). Below is one example of an (edited) proposal I received from Ricardo in which he explains his wish for a Council of Organizations to coordinate community organizing and improvement efforts in Marin City.

August 3, 2022

From: Ricardo Moncrief, ISOJI Director

RE: Council of Organizations (formerly Council of Agencies) for Marin City

To: Marin County social justice activists and social service agencies (including the Marin County Equity Implementation Team)

To whom it may concern,

At 80-years-of age, having been a community organizer in Marin County for approximately 20 years, I feel that my observations and insights are valuable toward realizing greater social equity in Marin County. I am putting my thoughts together in this document regarding what I believe to be a very important aspect that is missing from our efforts to improve life conditions for residents of Marin City, and more broadly, residents of Marin County.

I am happy to speak with you to answer any questions you may have.

Sincerely,
Ricardo Moncrief
hnef@aol.com

The Current Situation (the "Problem")

There have been attempts and alternate community building projects (e.g. Bolden, CSD's Community's Center of Life) in Marin City over the years which have been unsuccessful in reaching their goals (for various reasons). Importantly, there is no Marin City Integrated Masterplan.

A Brief History of Community Losses in Marin City

A lot has come and disappeared. There is a deep history and still we, along with the Canal (San Rafael) are the axis of California's worst disparities.

Marin City's losses include loss of lands, resources, complete service provers, flea markets, loss of political voice, increased gentrification (possibly annexation or incorporation), leading to greater unemployment, loss of community members who can't afford to stay, loss of concerts and other cultural events.

In 1999 when MCF withdrew its funding, there was a dismantling of all the previously successful local provider organizations that led MCF to get involved in the first place.

Coupled with racism, classism, divided community, diminished internal voices, no political power, no money, or fundraising mechanism, and no integrated plan, the community was "almost" barren of services . . . and hence, the emergence of ISOJI (e-so-gee) in 2000. This collective began a meek revitalization process focusing on education and the health and wellness center. Other initiatives followed.

The Desired Situation
Currently there are 10 decision-making entities or organizational voices. With the right type of facilitation these groups could create the type administrative and technical tools that have the potential to align multiple community and county interests.

My Suggested Path Forward
As the director of ISOJI, and speaking with participants of ISOJI, we have always felt the center of gravity for any community building effort (and in support of housing) is the Community Services District (CSD), our local government. But this should be aligned with and tied to a Community Council of Organizations. There are many reasons for this, including whole-community planning and technical oversight alignment with honest brokers and partnerships.

Some important components of a healthy, thriving community include the following:

- **Equity Build Pilot Program** for the County Implementation Team to consider as a special project
- **Community credit union** or banking/land management financial systems
- **Speaker's Bureau** – continuous learning and motivational efforts
- **Community Land Trust** – management of local lands (valuable)
- **Protocols for language barriers** and cross cultural (Latino) communications
- Funds allocated for **a skilled facilitator** or group leaders (and local facilitation training), along with an administrative technician with a possible extended staff and volunteer support. Technical consultants will also be needed to empower and coordinate the more technical systems.

Each of the items above are complex, multi-year projects. ISJOI was the birthplace of the Marin City Community Clinic; that was an enormous task that took several years and countless volunteer hours, in addition to funding and paid consultants, and we prevailed even in the face of a hostile local environment with people in powerful positions actively working against us. In short, I believe Marin City, with support from Marin County rather than opposition, is up to these crucial tasks.

What is At Stake

Marin City is on a cliff in terms of its survival as a community. It is a very small, low-income, under-resourced, culturally rich community that is situated on extraordinarily high value real estate. Having been predominantly African American in the past (approximately 70%) it is now approximately 38% African American, and one of, if not the most ethnically diverse community in an otherwise White county. If we don't get better organized as a community, i.e., create something like a Council of Organizations to come together for the benefit of all of us, Marin City will be gentrified. This will be a loss for all African American people who have a connection to Marin City, whether they still live in Marin County or not.

Council of Organizations Organizing Components (COO)

1. **Communications** — Increased intersectionality/ cross-sector communications, first between key agencies, agencies to constituencies, constituencies to families... community to County officials. Every agency/organization should know what the others are doing/planning at all times.

2. **Equity Reporting** — Establish and distribute an Equity Report Card or similar news/information recap of ongoing works, changes in the equity status ... possibly using baselines and progressive indicators... a visible display of growth and the narrowing or elimination of current disparities – oversee all incoming and outcoming data/images ... anything

that impacts public and community perceptions
and relations.

3. **Social and Print Media** — Use social media, news-
    letter, data/fact sheets, etc., via the postal service to
    distribute to "every" mailbox up-to-date informa-
    tion. We previously did this with the community
    newspaper "Marin City Today" – it went to every
    home and business (including the shopping center).
    The impact was visible.

4. **Political Unity/Strength** — Established political
    power/unity of a community voice through infra-
    structure cohesion, polices, outreach, community
    forums ... become a very visible part of the County
    planning decision making process ... COO should
    focus on political "parity" shared power with the
    County. The Supervisor can help achieve this
    objective.

5. **Economics** — Establish and implement economic
    priorities and contribute to economic priorities/
    communications and make note of wealth building,
    land and home ownership wherever possible. Please
    check out the missing role of **CDFI** "Community
    Development Financial Institutions" and/or banks/
    credit unions that can assist communities with these
    valuable institutions.

6. **Joint Proposals** — Author joint proposals or
    convene joint projects with a focus on "collective
    impacts" and the positive change in equity status.

7. **Image Building** is an ongoing deep concern and shouldn't be determined by negative social impacts that persist in people's minds.

8. **Race Counts** — Explore and document community implications and impact on the Race Counts reports. The county will have to adjust to this report because the level disparities emerging from Marin City is indisputable and must be addressed head-on if County statistics are going reflect change and growth.

9. **ART** — Use community ARTs and the Art-Is-Health movement to the fullest extent possible. Find pathways to honor internal voices. Use of the Art and Cultural Center is an invaluable asset in mobilizing voices of all ages and educational pedigree. See Oshalla, Felicia, Arts department at the school, Seniors, ISOJI, and others.

10. **Trust — Vital**: Work on policies that increase the "trust" relationship between decision-makers (e.g., local leaders), external providers, County decision makers, political officials and **especially developers** – higher levels of trust are critical because of the gradual erosion between leadership and especially developers (note the previous loss of lands and government revenues).

11. **Mental Health** — Support wrap-around mental health systems and the inclusion of the Family Function Scale to help track thriving families.

12. **Establish a fund-raising** mechanism/department or partnership, like a donor advised fund with MCF.

13. **Create a liaison** with County Planning Department/ community development.

14. Integrate and/or review **external grants** on behalf of the community, such as the ABAG. Activist just recently learned of a housing inspection committee that was trying to squeeze grant by community observers.

15. **Environmental Safety, Disaster Control, Health** — See Terrie H. Green.

16. **Support Government** — there should be an in-depth conversation regarding the supporting and clarification of the role of government.

ILLUSTRATION PERMISSIONS

Images were supplied courtesy of the author with the exception of the following.

FIG. 6. From "'Missing Meals' in Marin, San Francisco-Marin Food Bank 2019 Fact Sheet," https://www.sfmfoodbank.org/wp-content/uploads/2019/04/MM2019-FactSheet-MARIN_FINAL.pdf

FIG. 7. From https://www.cdc.gov/reproductivehealth/maternal-mortality/disparities-pregnancy-related-deaths/Infographic-disparities-pregnancy-related-deaths-h.pdf

FIG. 8. From page 30, https://www.chcf.org/wp-content/uploads/2019/11/MaternityCareCAAlmanac2019.pdf

FIG. 9. From https://insight.livestories.com/s/v2/chronic-diseasedashboard-marin-county/545a68f2-34bd-4ba6-a0f5-c2b3433a67fb/

FIG. 10. Modified from page 18, https://www.measureofamerica.org/docs/APOM_Final-SinglePages_12.14.11.pdf

FIG. 16. From https://statisticalatlas.com/county/California/Marin-County/Educational-Attainment#figure/educational-attainment-sex-ratio

FIG. 19, 20, 21. Modified from https://www.drought.gov/states/california/county/Marin

INDEX

www.ingramcontent.com/pod-product-compliance
Lightning Source LLC
Chambersburg PA
CBHW071735270326
41928CB00013B/2682